Risk Assessment in the Federal Government: Managing the Process

Committee on the Institutional Means for
Assessment of Risks to Public Health

Commission on Life Sciences

National Research Council

NATIONAL ACADEMY PRESS
Washington, D. C. 1983

The study reported here was supported by Contract
223-81-8251 between the National Academy of Sciences and
the Food and Drug Administration, Department of Health
and Human Services.

Library of Congress Catalog Card Number 83-80381

International Standard Book Number 0-309-03349-7

Available from:

NATIONAL ACADEMY PRESS
2101 Constitution Avenue, NW
Washington, D.C. 20418

Printed in the United States of America

March 1, 1983

Arthur Hull Hayes, Jr., M.D.
Commissioner of Food and Drugs
Food and Drug Administration
5600 Fishers Lane
Rockville, MD   20857

Dear Dr. Hayes:

   I am pleased to transmit the enclosed report entitled
"Risk Assessment in the Federal Government: Managing the
Process." This study was authorized by P.L. 96-528 and
carried out by a committee of the National Research
Council's Commission on Life Sciences with support from
the Food and Drug Administration under Contract No.
223-81-8251.

   The Congress made provision for this study to
strengthen the reliability and objectivity of scientific
assessment that forms the basis for federal regulatory
policies applicable to carcinogens and other public health
hazards. Federal agencies that perform risk assessments
are often hard pressed to clearly and convincingly present
the scientific basis for their regulatory decision. In
the recent past, for example, decisions on saccharin,
nitrites in food, formaldehyde use in home insulations,
asbestos, air pollutants and a host of other substances
have been called into question.

   The report recommends no radical changes in the
organizational arrangements for performing risk assessments. Rather, the committee finds that the basic problem
in risk assessment is the incompleteness of data, a
problem not remedied by changing the organizational
arrangement for performance of the assessments. Instead,
the committee has suggested a course of action to improve
the process within the practical constraints that exist.

THE NATIONAL RESEARCH COUNCIL IS THE PRINCIPAL OPERATING AGENCY OF THE NATIONAL ACADEMY OF SCIENCES AND THE NATIONAL ACADEMY OF ENGINEERING

TO SERVE GOVERNMENT AND OTHER ORGANIZATIONS.

One proposal by the committee requires explanation.
It would provide that there be established under Academy
auspices a Board on Risk Assessment Methods. This recommendation emerges strictly from the committee's internal
deliberation. The committee alone is responsible for the
substantive contents and findings of the report. Were a
request made to the Academy along the lines of that
particular recommendation to establish such a Board, the
request would be considered de novo by the appropriate
governing bodies of the institution.

Yours sincerely,

Frank Press
Chairman

Committee on the Institutional Means for Assessment of Risks to Public Health

REUEL A. STALLONES, School of Public Health, University
of Texas, Houston, Tex., Chairman
MORTON CORN, Department of Environmental Health Sciences,
Johns Hopkins University School of Hygiene and Public
Health, Baltimore, Md.
KENNY S. CRUMP, Science Research Systems, Inc., Ruston,
La.
J. CLARENCE DAVIES, Conservation Foundation, Washington,
D.C.
VINCENT P. DOLE, Rockefeller University, New York, N.Y.
TED R. I. GREENWOOD, Department of Political Science,
Massachusetts Institute of Technology, Cambridge, Mass.
RICHARD A. MERRILL, University of Virginia School of Law,
Charlottesville, Va.
FRANKLIN E. MIRER, Department of Health and Safety,
International Union, UAW, Detroit, Mich.
D. WARNER NORTH, Decision Focus, Inc., Los Altos, Calif.
GILBERT S. OMENN, Department of Environmental Health,
University of Washington School of Public Health and
Community Medicine, Seattle, Wash.
JOSEPH V. RODRICKS, ENVIRON Corporation, Washington, D.C.
PAUL SLOVIC, Decision Research, A Branch of
Perceptronics, Inc., Eugene, Oreg.
H. M. D. UTIDJIAN, American Cyanamid Company, Wayne, N.J.
ELIZABETH WEISBURGER, National Cancer Institute, National
Institutes of Health, Bethesda, Md.

Staff

LAWRENCE E. McCRAY, Project Director
CATHERINE L. ST. HILAIRE, Staff Officer
WILLIAM M. STIGLIANI, Staff Officer
RENEE M. ST. PIERRE, Administrative Secretary
NORMAN GROSSBLATT, Editor

Acknowledgments

The Committee acknowledges with appreciation information provided by the following persons.

KARIM AHMED, Research Director, Natural Resources Defense Council

ELIZABETH ANDERSON, Director, Office of Health and Environmental Assessment, Environmental Protection Agency

EDWIN L. BEHRENS, Procter and Gamble Corporation (representing American Industrial Health Council)

JACKSON B. BROWNING, Union Carbide Corporation (representing Chemical Manufacturers Association)

WILLIAM D. CAREY, Executive Officer, American Association for the Advancement of Science

PETER F. CARPENTER, Vice President for Corporate Strategy, Alza Corp., Palo Alto, Calif. (representing Pharmaceutical Manufacturers Association)

PAUL F. DEISLER, JR., Vice President, Health Safety and Environment, Shell Oil Company

ROBERT I. FIELD, Research Associate, Analysis and Inference, Inc., Boston, Mass.

W. GARY FLAMM, Deputy Associate Commissioner for Health Affairs (Science), Food and Drug Administration

SHERWIN GARDNER, Vice President, Science and Technology, Grocery Manufacturers of America, Inc.

MICHAEL GOUGH, Health Program Project Director, Office of Technology Assessment, U.S. Congress.

THOMAS P. GRUMBLY, Senior Consultant, Temple, Barker and Sloan, Inc., Lexington, Mass.

PAUL T. HOPPER, General Foods Corporation, (representing Social and Economic Committee, Food Safety Council)

NATHAN J. KARCH, Assistant Professor, Howard University; and Senior Science Advisor, Clement Associates

RAPHAEL G. KASPER, Executive Director, Commission on
    Physical Sciences, Mathematics, and Resources, NAS-NRC
ARNOLD M. KUZMACK, Chevy Chase, Md.
RICHARD LEMEN, Director, Division of Standards
    Development and Technology Transfer, National
    Institute of Occupational Safety and Health
JOHN MARTONIK, Deputy Director of Health Standards
    Programs, Occupational Safety and Health Administration
WILLIAM McCARVILLE, Monsanto Co., (representing American
    Industrial Health Council)
SANFORD A. MILLER, Director, Bureau of Foods, Food and
    Drug Administration.
PAUL MILVY, Environmental Law Institute
WARREN R. MUIR, Visiting Associate Professor, Department
    of Environmental Sciences, Johns Hopkins University
DENIS PRAGER, Assistant Director for Life Sciences and
    Institutional Relations, Office of Science and
    Technology Policy, Executive Office of the President
PETER PREUSS, Associate Executive Director, Directorate
    of Health Sciences, Consumer Product Safety Commission
DAVID RALL, Director, National Institute of Environmental
    Health Sciences
WILLIAM D. ROWE, Director, Institute for Risk Analysis;
    and Professor of Decision and Risk Analysis, American
    University
JAMES H. SAMMONS, Executive Vice President, American
    Medical Association
SHELDON SAMUELS, Director, Health Safety and
    Environmental Industrial Union Department, AFL/CIO
BRUCE SILVERGLADE, Director for Legal Affairs, Center for
    Science in the Public Interest
M. J. SLOAN, Manager, Regulatory Affairs, Shell Oil
    Company
STEVEN M. SWANSON, Director, Health and Safety
    Regulation, American Petroleum Institute
ROBERT G. TARDIFF, Executive Director, Board on
    Toxicology and Environmental Health Hazards, NAS-NRC
MONTE C. THRODAHL, Monsanto Corporation (representing
    American Industrial Health Council)
HAROLD TRABOSH, Deputy Director, Residue Evaluation and
    Surveillance Division, Food Safety Inspection Service,
    Department of Agriculture
REP. WILLIAM C. WAMPLER (D-VA), U.S. House of
    Representatives

Preface

In response to a directive from the Congress of the United States, the Food and Drug Administration contracted with the National Academy of Sciences to conduct a study of the institutional means for risk assessment. The Committee on the Institutional Means for Assessment of Risks to Public Health was formed in the National Research Council's Commission on Life Sciences in October 1981 and completed its work in January 1983. The members of the Committee were chosen to represent a broad array of backgrounds and special skills, both in the technology of risk assessment and in the formulation and application of policy in this field, and brought together extensive experience in industry, government, and academic life.

The Committee, with outstanding staff support, reviewed much of the published literature on risk assessment, studied the structures and operations of federal regulatory and research agencies, analyzed the history of regulation of selected chemicals, and sought and received the judgments of some exceptionally knowledgeable people. We are most grateful for the assistance so generously provided to us, but, of course, the responsibility for this report is entirely ours.

The Committee has sought to examine and codify past experience with risk assessment and relate that experience to patterns and practices. Our judgments are necessarily subjective, but we have endeavored to be impartial. In the process, we developed a disinclination for sweeping changes; we believe that more gradual, evolutionary alterations will result in greater improvements in the conduct and use of risk assessment.

REUEL A. STALLONES
Chairman

Contents

Risk Assessment in the Federal Government: Managing the Process

Summary

SETTING

This report explores the intricate relations between science and policy in a field that is the subject of much debate--the assessment of the risk of cancer and other adverse health effects associated with exposure of humans to toxic substances. It is a report of a search for the institutional mechanisms that best foster a constructive partnership between science and government, mechanisms to ensure that government regulation rests on the best available scientific knowledge and to preserve the integrity of scientific data and judgments in the unavoidable collision of the contending interests that accompany most important regulatory decisions.

Many decisions of federal agencies in regulating chronic health hazards have been bitterly controversial. The roots of the controversy lie in improvements in scientific and technologic capability to detect potentially hazardous chemicals, in changes in public expectations and concerns about health protection, and in the fact that the costs and benefits of regulatory policies fall unequally on different groups within American society.

The decade of the 1970s was a period of heightened public concern about the effects of technology on the environment. Individuals and groups urged strict government regulation as scientific evidence emerged that various chemical substances may induce cancers or other chronic health effects in humans, and new government programs were established to control potential hazards. The evidence of health effects of a few chemicals, such as asbestos, has been clear; in many more cases the evidence is meager and indirect. To aid decision-making,

1

agencies have developed procedures for identifying chronic health hazards and estimating the risks to human health posed by products and activities. However, rather than alleviating the controversy attending regulatory decisions, the procedures themselves have become a focus of criticism by scientists, industry representatives, and public-interest groups.

STUDY OBJECTIVES AND SCOPE

The Committee on Institutional Means for Assessment of Risks to Public Health was formed, in response to a congressional directive, to fulfill three primary objectives:

- To assess the merits of separating the analytic functions of developing risk assessments from the regulatory functions of making policy decisions.
- To consider the feasibility of designating a single organization to do risk assessments for all regulatory agencies.
- To consider the feasibility of developing uniform risk assessment guidelines for use by all regulatory agencies.

The Committee considered the current practice of risk assessment and its relation to the process of regulation of hazards to human health, past efforts to develop and use risk assessment guidelines, the experience of government regulatory agencies with different administrative arrangements for risk assessment, and various proposals to modify risk assessment procedures. Our study was directed primarily, although not exclusively, to the issue of increased risk of cancer resulting from exposure to chemicals in the environment, an issue that has aroused great public concern in recent years, as illustrated by the controversies involving the control of saccharin, asbestos, and formaldehyde. Despite this emphasis, however, our conclusions and recommendations are applicable in some degree across the broad field of environmental health.

Criticisms of risk assessment have ranged broadly from details of the process to administrative management to statutory authority. The mandate to this Committee did not include examination of the scientific issues involved in risk assessment or the broad social policy questions

that have been raised. The Committee's more limited
purpose was to examine whether altered <u>institutional
arrangements or procedures</u> can improve regulatory
performance.

THE NATURE OF RISK ASSESSMENT

Regulatory actions are based on two distinct elements,
<u>risk assessment,</u> the subject of this study, and <u>risk
management.</u> Risk assessment is the use of the factual
base to define the health effects of exposure of individuals or populations to hazardous materials and situations. Risk management is the process of weighing
policy alternatives and selecting the most appropriate
regulatory action, integrating the results of risk
assessment with engineering data and with social,
economic, and political concerns to reach a decision.
  Risk assessments contain some or all of the following
four steps:

  • <u>Hazard identification</u>: The determination of
whether a particular chemical is or is not causally
linked to particular health effects.
  • <u>Dose-response assessment</u>: The determination of
the relation between the magnitude of exposure and the
probability of occurrence of the health effects in
question.
  • <u>Exposure assessment</u>: The determination of the
extent of human exposure before or after application of
regulatory controls.
  • <u>Risk characterization</u>: The description of the
nature and often the magnitude of human risk, including
attendant uncertainty.

  In each step, a number of decision points (<u>components</u>)
occur where risk to human health can only be inferred
from the available evidence. Both scientific judgments
and policy choices may be involved in selecting from
among possible inferential bridges, and we have used the
term <u>risk assessment policy</u> to differentiate those judgments and choices from the broader social and economic
policy issues that are inherent in risk management decisions. At least some of the controversy surrounding
regulatory actions has resulted from a blurring of the
distinction between risk assessment policy and risk
management policy.

UNIFORM GUIDELINES FOR RISK ASSESSMENT

An _inference guideline_ is an explicit statement of a pre-determined choice among alternative methods (_inference options_) that might be used to infer human risk from data that are not fully adequate or are not drawn directly from human experience. For example, a guideline might specify the mathematical model to be used to estimate the effects of exposure at low doses on the basis of the effects of exposure at high doses.

Over the last 2 decades, most federal regulatory agencies and other institutions responsible for risk assessment of toxic chemicals have sought to develop such guidelines. Their efforts have met with varied success. Agencies have cited several reasons for writing guidelines: to provide a systematic way to meet statutory requirements, to inform the public and regulated industries of agency policies, to stimulate public comment on those policies, to avoid arguing generic questions anew in each specific case, and to foster consistency and continuity of approach. Interagency guidelines for carcinogens, although short-lived, were developed by the agencies of the Interagency Regulatory Liaison Group (IRLG) and adopted by the President's Regulatory Council in 1979. The stated objective of that effort was to reduce inconsistency, duplication of effort, and lack of coordination among the federal agencies.

The form of guidelines varies widely. Some guidelines are comprehensive and detailed, addressing most of the components of risk assessment and describing underlying scientific concepts; others address only a few broad principles. Guidelines differ greatly in their degree of flexibility, i.e., the degree to which they permit assessors to consider scientific evidence that may justify departures from the prescribed inference options. And they vary in the legal authority vested in them: some are adopted as formal regulations and others by less formal means.

The Committee concludes that guidelines are feasible and, if properly designed, desirable; that clear statements of the inferences to be made in each step would be of advantage to the regulatory agencies, to the industries concerned, and to the general public; and that guidelines should be used uniformly by the governmental agencies.

INSTITUTIONAL ARRANGEMENTS FOR RISK ASSESSMENT

Dissatisfaction with government regulatory actions has led to proposals to restructure the institutional arrangements for risk assessment by:

* Organizational separation of risk assessment from risk management.
* Centralization of risk assessment activities in a single organization to serve all the regulatory agencies.

Four federal agencies--the Environmental Protection Agency (EPA), Food and Drug Administration (FDA), Occupational Safety and Health Administration (OSHA), and Consumer Product Safety Commission (CPSC)--have been given primary authority to regulate activities and substances that pose chronic health risks, and these four agencies' past actions have inspired many of the proposals for institutional change. The Committee reviewed a number of agency structures and procedures in an attempt to determine the merits of institutional separation and centralization. Examples were selected to illustrate different degrees of separation and centralization in the four agencies. Independent scientific review panels have been used to obtain some of the advantages proposed for organizational separation, and some of their experiences were examined.

Cross-agency comparisons are difficult, because the regulatory agencies and their various programs differ markedly in structure, procedures, personnel characteristics, administrative history, and statutory direction. In addition, agencies and programs change, and practices adhered to for several years may be altered substantially. These practical limitations to the evaluation of agency structures and practices led the Committee to conclude that predicting the likely effects of organizational rearrangements on agency performance of risk assessment is unavoidably judgmental. However, the available evidence shows no clear advantage of one administrative structure over another.

CONCLUSIONS AND MAJOR RECOMMENDATIONS

Dissatisfaction with the actions of federal regulatory agencies is often expressed as criticism of the conduct and administration of the risk assessment process. The

Committee believes that the basic problem in risk assessment is the sparseness and uncertainty of the scientific knowledge of the health hazards addressed, and this problem has no ready solution. The field has been developing rapidly, and the greatest improvements in risk assessment result from the acquisition of more and better data, which decreases the need to rely on inference and informed judgment to bridge gaps in knowledge.

Proposals to separate the administrative responsibility for risk assessment from risk management imply that the change would lead to improved risk assessment and hence better risk management decisions. Administrative relocation will not, however, improve the knowledge base, and, because risk assessment is only one element in the formulation of regulatory actions, even considerable improvements in risk assessment cannot be expected to eliminate controversy over those actions.

Organizational separation may have the advantage of establishing firmly the distinction between risk assessment and risk management, but it also has some disadvantages. The importance of distinguishing between risk assessment and risk management does not imply that they should be isolated from each other; in practice they interact, and communication in both directions is desirable and should not be disrupted. Institutional separation would surely reduce the responsiveness of the risk assessment process to the needs of the regulatory agencies for timely reports in accord with their priorities. In addition to the operational disadvantages, the disruption of current patterns of activity would be great, and the benefits uncertain. On balance, the Committee believes that transfer of risk assessment functions to an organization separate from the regulatory agencies is not appropriate.

We believe that risk assessment can be improved more surely and more effectively by adopting a program with three major parts: (A) implementation of procedural changes to ensure that individual assessments routinely take full advantage of the available scientific knowledge, while preserving the diversified approaches to the administration of risk assessment necessary to accommodate the varied needs of federal regulatory programs; (B) standardization of analytic procedures among federal programs through the development and use of uniform inference guidelines; and (C) creation of a mechanism that will ensure orderly and continuing review and modification of

risk assessment procedures as the scientific knowledge
base expands.

(A) <u>We recommend that regulatory agencies take steps
to establish and maintain a clear conceptual
distinction between assessment of risks and consideration of risk management alternatives; that is, the
scientific findings and policy judgments embodied in
risk assessments should be explicitly distinguished
from the political, economic, and technical
considerations that influence the design and choice of
regulatory strategies.</u>

We agree with proponents of such measures as the
American Industrial Health Council's proposed science
panel and H.R. 638 that efforts should be made by regulators and others to distinguish clearly between the
assessment of risk and the choice of regulatory options.
We advocate the adoption of specific procedural measures that can be introduced under current arrangements.
These measures include timely independent scientific
review of major agency risk assessments and, to facilitate both scientific and public review of risk assessments, the routine preparation of written risk assessments that explicitly state the basis of choice among
inference options.

(B) <u>We recommend that uniform inference guidelines be developed for the use of federal regulatory agencies in the risk assessment process.</u>

The Committee endorses the development and use of
guidelines for risk assessment. These guidelines, which
would structure the interpretation of scientific and technical information relevant to the assessment of health
risks, should be followed by all federal agencies. They
should address all elements of risk assessment, but allow
flexibility to consider unique scientific evidence in
particular instances.
The use of uniform guidelines would promote clarity,
completeness, and consistency in risk assessment; would
clarify the relative roles of scientific and other factors
in risk assessment policy; would help to ensure that
assessments reflect the latest scientific understanding;
and would enable regulated parties to anticipate government decisions. In addition, adherence to inference

guidelines will aid in maintaining the distinction between risk assessment and risk management.

(C) We recommend to the Congress that a Board on Risk Assessment Methods be established to perform the following functions:
  (1) To assess critically the evolving scientific basis of risk assessment and to make explicit the underlying assumptions and policy ramifications of the inference options in each component of the risk assessment process.
  (2) To draft and periodically to revise recommended inference guidelines for risk assessment for adoption and use by federal regulatory agencies.
  (3) To study agency experience with risk assessment and evaluate the usefulness of the guidelines.
  (4) To identify research needs in the risk assessment field and in relevant underlying disciplines.

The Committee concludes that success in improving the risk assessment process requires the establishment of an independent board of scientific stature. Such a board can serve as a continuing locus of discussion about ways to improve scientific and procedural aspects of risk assessment.

Introduction

Through Congress the American public has granted authority to federal administrative agencies to restrict private
actions, such as the production and use of chemicals,
when this is deemed necessary to protect the health of
the public. The 1970s are notable for the large number
of new federal regulatory laws that are applicable to the
environment, both in the workplace and in the community.
These laws reflect a dramatic and relatively rapid shift
in public priorities toward the protection of health.
Concurrently with shifts in social priorities, advances
in science have contributed to policy problems, for the
advances have revealed the extent of the environmental
health problem. Some earlier regulatory programs had
addressed exposure to toxic chemicals, but they were
directed mainly at the risk of poisoning and other acute
effects. Much policy-making related to such effects
involved routine, short-term, acute animal studies to
establish "no-observed-effect" doses and then the
straightforward calculation of allowable human exposure
based on the application of safety factors to relatively
uncomplicated scientific findings. Such an approach
reflected little recognition of problems that might be
associated with smaller exposures. Cancer, birth defects,
and other conditions were seldom seen as preventable by
government intervention. Only in the last 15 years has
the potential extent of the linkage between such conditions and toxic substances been revealed. The often-
cited estimate that a large fraction of all cancers may
be attributed to human exposure to toxic agents (including
smoking, diet, lifestyle, and occupation) originated
fairly recently (Boyland, 1969; Higginson, 1969), and it

was not until the 1970s that regulatory agencies focused their attention on cancer and other chronic health risks.

Scientific advances entered the picture in a second way. The technology that has made it possible to detect relations between particular agents and cancer or other chronic effects has evolved rapidly from the days when exposure through skin-painting and subcutaneous injection were relied on in animal tests of carcinogenicity. Increasingly, epidemiologic investigations have either confirmed the findings of animal experiments or provided evidence that linked exposures to particular chemicals to particular chronic health effects. The introduction of reliable testing methods resulted in broader government testing requirements and, steadily, the discovery of more and more suspect chemicals—many of them in common use—that demanded agency attention. The techniques are still developing, and we are still looking for better ways to design and interpret animal bioassay experiments.

The increase in newly suspect chemicals was accompanied by the development of instruments and procedures that permitted the detection of chemicals at lower and lower concentrations. Even if the number of suspect chemicals had not increased dramatically, these sensitive detection methods would have revealed the presence of such chemicals in concentrations that earlier methods would have missed. Combined with all those changes were the development and refinement of analytic methods of estimating the degree of human risk on the basis of data from human studies and animal experiments.

Public policies are not immediately adaptable to rapid changes in social priorities and scientific advances. Many of the fundamental difficulties of regulatory risk assessment result from attempts to bend old laws and policies to fit newly perceived risks. For instance:

• A regulatory framework based on the traditional approach involving no-observed-effect doses and safety factors is now being applied to health effects for which a no-effect dose cannot be demonstrated, except at zero exposure.

• Regulatory laws and programs designed for the elimination of what was understood to be the very rare event of chronic hazard now operate in the presence of the recognition that many agents are suspect.

• Agencies must evaluate hundreds of chemicals on which no data related to human risk are available and on

which few animal tests were required and many other
chemicals that were tested with methods that do not meet
modern standards.
  • Laws were written and programs designed before
current quantitative methods for estimating human risks
on the basis of data from animal studies were developed.

DIFFICULTIES IN DECISION-MAKING

Agency decisions regarding potential carcinogens and
similar hazards are commonly beset by two types of difficulties: inherent limitations on the power of analysis
and practical constraints imposed by external pressures.
Several such factors are particularly relevant to the
consideration of scientific aspects of risk assessment.

INHERENT LIMITATIONS

Uncertainty

The dominant analytic difficulty is pervasive uncertainty.
Risk assessment draws extensively on science, and a strong
scientific basis has developed for linking exposure to
chemicals to chronic health effects. However, data may
be incomplete, and there is often great uncertainty in
estimates of the types, probability, and magnitude of
health effects associated with a chemical agent, of the
economic effects of a proposed regulatory action, and of
the extent of current and possible future human exposures.
These problems have no immediate solutions, given the
many gaps in our understanding of the causal mechanisms
of carcinogenesis and other health effects and in our
ability to ascertain the nature or extent of the effects
associated with specific exposures. Because our knowledge
is limited, conclusive direct evidence of a threat to
human health is rare. Fewer than 30 agents are definitely
linked with cancer in humans (Tomatis et al., 1978); in
contrast, some 1,500 substances are reportedly carcinogenic in animal tests, although they include substances
tested in studies of questionable experimental design.
We know even less about most chemicals; only about 7,000
of the over 5,000,000 known substances have ever been
tested for carcinogenicity (Maugh, 1978)--a small fraction
of those theoretically under regulatory jurisdiction. We

know still less about chronic health effects other than cancer.

Ethical considerations prevent deliberate human experimentation with potentially dangerous chemicals, and the length of the latent period for cancer and some other effects greatly complicates epidemiologic studies of uncontrolled human exposures. Animal models must be used to investigate whether exposure to a chemical is related to the incidence of health effects, and the results must be extrapolated to humans. To make judgments amid such uncertainty, risk assessors must rely on a series of assumptions.

Limited Analytic Resources

The number of chemicals in the jurisdiction of federal regulatory agencies is enormous. For example, of the roughly 5,000,000 known chemicals, more than 70,000 are in commercial use (Fishbein, 1980). The Environmental Protection Agency's Chemical Activities Status Report lists about 3,500 chemicals as being under some sort of active consideration in the Agency's various regulatory programs. Similarly, the Food and Drug Administration's food program must cope with over 2,000 food-related chemicals (900 flavors, 700 items listed as "generally recognized as safe," 350 food additives, 175 animal drugs, and 60 color additives) and an additional 12,000 indirect additives (Flamm, 1981).

The many problem chemicals in an agency's jurisdiction compete for attention of analysts and decision-makers. If an agency is considering new action on many substances at once, its scientific staff is stretched thin. Most agencies do not have the analytic resources to do a thorough risk assessment for priority-setting and must rely on less formal methods to ensure that the highest-risk chemicals are examined first.

Complexity

For most chemical agents that might be subject to regulation, a great variety of factors must be assessed, including potential toxicity, extent of human exposure, effectiveness of technologies to reduce exposure, the nature of possible substitute chemicals, effects on and interests of various population groups, and economic effects of

regulatory alternatives. Decision-makers in a regulatory
agency may encounter a large amount of highly technical
information as they work toward their decisions; many
scientific disciplines and technical fields are usually
involved. An agency would like to have simple rules and
analytic procedures to ensure consistency and competence
in its decision-making, but, in the face of scientific
uncertainty, such simplicity is difficult to achieve
without an inadvertent loss of crucial scientific insight
from the decision process.

EXTERNAL PRESSURES

Public Concern with Health Protection

When the risk involves a serious disease, such as cancer,
or birth defects, feelings are likely to run high, particularly if the groups exposed to a chemical are mobil-
ized to express themselves in an agency's deliberations.
Such groups insist that regulatory action need not await
conclusive evidence of cause and effect and need not be
based exclusively on the most scientifically advanced
testing methods.

Visible Economic Interests

Although it is rarely known which individuals are likely
to be saved from adverse health effects through a regulation that reduces exposure to a particular chemical,
those who bear the economic costs of such restrictions
can identify themselves without any difficulty. These
parties can provide relatively concrete projections of a
prospective regulation's inflationary influence, effect
on employment, and other immediate economic effects, and
such consequences may be substantial. They may question
the wisdom of balancing concrete evidence of economic
damage against evidence of health protection that depends
on a complex series of assumptions derived from sparse
and indirect data.

Congressional Action

In fulfilling its role as the legislative voice of popular
concerns, Congress can act in ways that influence decision

processes. It can dictate the factors to be included in and excluded from decision-making (the Delaney clause is an example), and it can pass special legislation to pre-empt agency discretion, as it did in acting to prevent the removal of saccharin from the market.

PROPOSED REFORMS

Under these conditions, it would perhaps be surprising if calls for major reform were not heard. Some have sought to improve the techniques that the government uses to analyze and evaluate risks; for example, the House of Representatives in 1982 passed H.R. 6159 (commonly known as the "Ritter bill"), to establish a government-wide program of research and demonstration projects on quantitative and comparative risk analysis.

Much of the recent controversy is general; it reflects the conflict in values between different groups in society, particularly with regard to the relative importance of economic factors and health protection in the formulation of regulatory decisions. Different groups will inevitably disagree about the degree of risk (if any) that is defined as acceptable in a particular case. However, some criticisms directly address the risk assessment component of the overall decision-making process. Some critics question whether current practices adequately safeguard the quality of the scientific interpretations needed for risk assessment. With a scientific base that is still evolving, with large uncertainties to be addressed in each decision, and with the presence of great external pressures, some see a danger that the scientific interpretations in risk assessments will be distorted by policy considerations, and they seek new institutional safeguards against such distortion.

Among the institutional reforms suggested, two major categories are the focus of this report: reorganization to ensure that risk assessments are protected from inappropriate policy influences and development and use of uniform guidelines for carrying out risk assessments.

Some argue that scientific quality, consistency, and distinction between scientific judgment and policy judgment can be improved through the use of explicit guidelines for agency risk assessments. Such guidelines would specify methods for interpreting scientific data and would seek to limit analysts who confront data gaps or extrapolation questions to methods that are consistent with the best current scientific judgment. Analysts following the guidelines would find it easier to describe systematically and explicitly the methods that are incorporated in their risk assessments.

Several other recent proposals call for major restructuring of federal processes to separate the risk assessment function organizationally from decision-making. The objectives would be to permit analysts to work independently of policy pressures and to foster consistency of risk assessments. Various approaches have been suggested, including creation of a single body outside the government for the performance or review of risk assessments, creation of a single government unit to conduct risk assessments for the entire government, and creation of separate risk assessment units in particular programs or agencies and systematic review of assessments by independent scientific advisory groups.

THE STUDY

This report responds to a congressional request to examine the merits of the two major types of reform proposal. It is the final report of the National Research Council's Committee on the Institutional Means for Assessment of Risks to Public Health. Chapter I describes the structure of risk assessment, the role of science in the assessment process, and current federal uses of risk assessment. Chapter II examines the feasibility and desirability of the development and use of uniform guidelines. Chapter III reviews various organizational arrangements for risk assessment. The Committee's overall conclusions and recommendations appear in Chapter IV.

REFERENCES

Boyland, E. 1969. The correlation of experimental carcinogenesis and cancer in man. Prog. Exp. Tumor Res. 77:222-234.

Fishbein, L. 1980. Potential industrial carcinogenic and mutagenic alkylating agents, pp. 329-363. In D. B. Walters, ed. Safe Handling of Chemical Carcinogens, Mutagens, Teratogens, and Highly Toxic Substances, vol. I. Ann Arbor, Mich.: Ann Arbor Science.

Flamm, W. G. October 13, 1981. Remarks to the Committee on the Institutional Means for Assessment of Risks to Public Health.

Higginson, J. 1969. Present trends in cancer epidemiology. In Proc. Can. Cancer Conf. 8:40-75.

Maugh, T. 1978. Who chooses chemicals for testing? Science 201:1200.

Tomatis, L., C. Agthe, H. Bartsch, J. Huff, R. Montesano, R. Saracci, E. Walker, and J. Wilbourn. 1978. Evaluation of the carcinogenicity of chemicals: a review of the monograph program of I.A.R.C. Cancer Res. 38:877.

I
The Nature of Risk Assessment

Recent criticisms of the conduct and use of risk assessment by regulatory agencies have led to a wide range of proposed remedies, including changes in regulatory statutes and the development of new methods for assessing risk. The mandate to this Committee was more limited. Our objective was to examine whether alterations in institutional arrangements or procedures, particularly the organizational separation of risk assessment from regulatory decision-making and the use of uniform guidelines for inferring risk from available scientific information, can improve federal risk assessment activities.

Before undertaking to determine whether organizational and procedural reforms could improve the performance and use of risk assessment in the federal government, the Committee examined the state of risk assessment and the regulatory environment in which it is performed. In this chapter, we define risk assessment and differentiate it from other elements in the regulatory process, analyze the types of judgments made in risk assessment, and examine its current government context. Because one chronic health hazard, cancer, was highlighted in the Committee's congressional mandate and has dominated public concern about public health risks in recent years, most of our report focuses on it. Furthermore, because activities in four agencies--the Environmental Protection Agency (EPA), the Food and Drug Administration (FDA), the Occupational Safety and Health Administration (OSHA), and the Consumer Product Safety Commission (CPSC)--have given rise to many of the proposals for changes in risk assessment practices, our review focuses on these four agencies. The conclusions of this report, although directed primarily at risk assessment of potential carcinogens as performed by these

four agencies, may be applicable to other federal programs
to reduce health risks.

TERMINOLOGY

Despite the fact that risk assessment has become a subject
that has been extensively discussed in recent years, no
standard definitions have evolved, and the same concepts
are encountered under different names. The Committee
adopted the following terminology for use in this report.

RISK ASSESSMENT AND RISK MANAGEMENT

We use risk assessment to mean the characterization of
the potential adverse health effects of human exposures
to environmental hazards. Risk assessments include
several elements: description of the potential adverse
health effects based on an evaluation of results of
epidemiologic, clinical, toxicologic, and environmental
research; extrapolation from those results to predict the
type and estimate the extent of health effects in humans
under given conditions of exposure; judgments as to the
number and characteristics of persons exposed at various
intensities and durations; and summary judgments on the
existence and overall magnitude of the public-health
problem. Risk assessment also includes characterization
of the uncertainties inherent in the process of inferring
risk.

The term risk assessment is often given narrower and
broader meanings than we have adopted here. For some
observers, the term is synonymous with quantitative risk
assessment and emphasizes reliance on numerical results.
Our broader definition includes quantification, but also
includes qualitative expressions of risk. Quantitative
estimates of risk are not always feasible, and they may
be eschewed by agencies for policy reasons. Broader uses
of the term than ours also embrace analysis of perceived
risks, comparisons of risks associated with different
regulatory strategies, and occasionally analysis of the
economic and social implications of regulatory decisions--
functions that we assign to risk management.

The Committee uses the term risk management to describe
the process of evaluating alternative regulatory actions
and selecting among them. Risk management, which is carried out by regulatory agencies under various legislative

mandates, is an agency decision-making process that
entails consideration of political, social, economic, and
engineering information with risk-related information to
develop, analyze, and compare regulatory options and to
select the appropriate regulatory response to a potential
chronic health hazard. The selection process necessarily
requires the use of value judgments on such issues as the
acceptability of risk and the reasonableness of the costs
of control.

STEPS IN RISK ASSESSMENT

Risk assessment can be divided into four major steps:
hazard identification, dose-response assessment, exposure
assessment, and risk characterization. A risk assessment
might stop with the first step, hazard identification, if
no adverse effect is found or if an agency elects to take
regulatory action without further analysis, for reasons
of policy or statutory mandate.

Of the four steps, hazard identification is the most
easily recognized in the actions of regulatory agencies.
It is defined here as the process of determining whether
exposure to an agent can cause an increase in the incidence of a health condition (cancer, birth defect, etc.).
It involves characterizing the nature and strength of the
evidence of causation. Although the question of whether
a substance causes cancer or other adverse health effects
is theoretically a yes-no question, there are few chemicals on which the human data are definitive. Therefore,
the question is often restated in terms of effects in
laboratory animals or other test systems, e.g., "Does the
agent induce cancer in test animals?" Positive answers
to such questions are typically taken as evidence that an
agent may pose a cancer risk for any exposed humans.
Information from short-term in vitro tests and on structural similarity to known chemical hazards may also be
considered.

Dose-response assessment is the process of characterizing the relation between the dose of an agent administered or received and the incidence of an adverse health
effect in exposed populations and estimating the incidence
of the effect as a function of human exposure to the
agent. It takes account of intensity of exposure, age
pattern of exposure, and possibly other variables that
might affect response, such as sex, lifestyle, and other
modifying factors. A dose-response assessment usually

requires extrapolation from high to low dose and extrapolation from animals to humans. A dose-response assessment should describe and justify the methods of extrapolation used to predict incidence and should characterize
the statistical and biologic uncertainties in these
methods.

    Exposure assessment is the process of measuring or
estimating the intensity, frequency, and duration of
human exposures to an agent currently present in the
environment or of estimating hypothetical exposures that
might arise from the release of new chemicals into the
environment. In its most complete form, it describes the
magnitude, duration, schedule, and route of exposure; the
size, nature, and classes of the human populations
exposed; and the uncertainties in all estimates. Exposure
assessment is often used to identify feasible prospective
control options and to predict the effects of available
control technologies on exposure.

    Risk characterization is the process of estimating the
incidence of a health effect under the various conditions
of human exposure described in exposure assessment. It
is performed by combining the exposure and dose-response
assessments. The summary effects of the uncertainties in
the preceding steps are described in this step.

    The relations among the four steps of risk assessment
and between risk assessment and risk management are
depicted in Figure I-1. The type of research information
needed for each step is also illustrated.

SCIENTIFIC BASIS FOR RISK ASSESSMENT

Step 1. Hazard Identification

Although risk assessment as it is currently practiced by
federal agencies for the estimation of carcinogenic risk
contains several relatively new features, the scientific
basis for much of the analysis done in risk assessment is
well established. This is especially true of the first
step in the assessment process, hazard identification.
Four general classes of information may be used in this
step: epidemiologic data, animal-bioassay data, data on
in vitro effects, and comparisons of molecular structure.

    Epidemiologic Data
    Well-conducted epidemiologic studies that show a posi-
tive association between an agent and a disease are

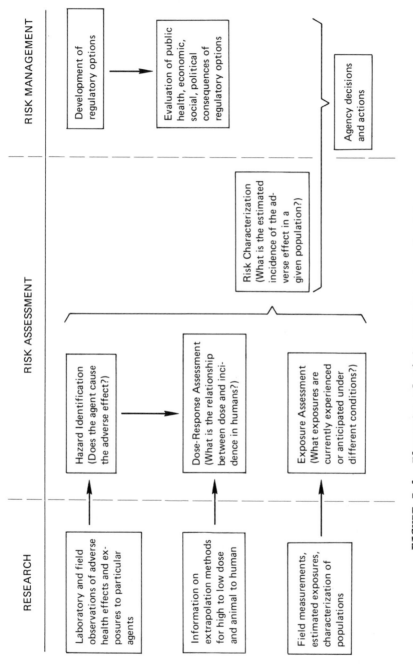

FIGURE I-1 Elements of risk assessment and risk management.

accepted as the most convincing evidence about human risk. This evidence is, however, difficult to accumulate; often the risk is low, the number of persons exposed is small, the latent period between exposure and disease is long, and exposures are mixed and multiple. Thus, epidemiologic data require careful interpretation. Even if these problems are solved satisfactorily, the preponderance of chemicals in the environment has not been studied with epidemiologic methods, and we would not wish to release newly produced substances only to discover years later that they were powerful carcinogenic agents. These limitations require reliance on less direct evidence that a health hazard exists.

Animal-Bioassay Data

The most commonly available data in hazard identification are those obtained from animal bioassays. The inference that results from animal experiments are applicable to humans is fundamental to toxicologic research; this premise underlies much of experimental biology and medicine and is logically extended to the experimental observation of carcinogenic effects. Despite the apparent validity of such inferences and their acceptability by most cancer researchers, there are no doubt occasions in which observations in animals may be of highly uncertain relevance to humans.

Consistently positive results in the two sexes and in several strains and species and higher incidences at higher doses constitute the best evidence of carcinogenicity. More often than not, however, such data are not available. Instead, because of the nature of the effect and the limits of detection of animal tests as they are usually conducted, experimental data leading to a positive finding sometimes barely exceed a statistical threshold and may involve tumor types of uncertain relation to human carcinogenesis. Interpretation of some animal data may therefore be difficult. Notwithstanding uncertainties associated with interpretation of some animal tests, they have, in general, proved to be reliable indicators of carcinogenic properties and will continue to play a pivotal role in efforts to identify carcinogens.

Short-Term Studies

Considerable experimental evidence supports the proposition that most chemical carcinogens are mutagens and that many mutagens are carcinogens. As a result, a positive response in a mutagenicity assay is supportive

evidence that the agent tested is likely to be carcinogenic. Such data, in the absence of a positive animal
bioassay, are rarely, if ever, sufficient to support a
conclusion that an agent is carcinogenic. Because short-
term tests are rapid and inexpensive, they are valuable
for screening chemicals for potential carcinogenicity and
lending additional support to observations from animal
and epidemiologic investigations.

Comparisons of Molecular Structure

Comparison of an agent's chemical or physical properties with those of known carcinogens provides some evidence of potential carcinogenicity. Experimental data
support such associations for a few structural classes;
however, such studies are best used to identify potential
carcinogens for further investigation and may be useful
in priority-setting for carcinogenicity testing.

Step 2. Dose-Response Assessment

In a small number of instances, epidemiologic data permit
a dose-response relation to be developed directly from
observations of exposure and health effects in humans.
If epidemiologic data are available, extrapolations from
the exposures observed in the study to lower exposures
experienced by the general population are often necessary.
Such extrapolations introduce uncertainty into the estimates of risk for the general population. Uncertainties
also arise because the general population includes some
people, such as children, who may be more susceptible
than people in the sample from which the epidemiologic
data were developed.

The absence of useful human data is common for most
chemicals being assessed for carcinogenic effect, and
dose-response assessment usually entails evaluating tests
that were performed on rats or mice. The tests, however,
typically have been designed for hazard identification,
rather than for determining dose-response relations.
Under current testing practice, one group of animals is
given the highest dose that can be tolerated, a second
group is exposed at half that dose, and a control group
is not exposed. (The use of high doses is necessary to
maximize the sensitivity of the study for determining
whether the agent being tested has carcinogenic potential.) A finding in such studies that increased exposure
leads to an increased incidence has been used primarily

to corroborate hazard identification, that is, to show that the agent does indeed induce the adverse health effect.

The testing of chemicals at high doses has been challenged by some scientists who argue that metabolism of chemicals differs at high and low doses; i.e., high doses may overwhelm normal detoxification mechanisms and provide results that would not occur at the lower doses to which humans are exposed. An additional factor that is often raised to challenge the validity of animal data to indicate effects in man is that metabolic differences among animal species should be considered when animal test results are analyzed. Metabolic differences can have important effects on the validity of extrapolating from animals to man if, for example, the actual carcinogen is a metabolite of the administered chemical and the animals tested differ markedly from humans in their production of that metabolite. A related point is that the actual dose of carcinogen reaching the affected tissue or organ is usually not known; thus, dose-response information, of necessity, is based on administered dose and not tissue dose. Although data of these types would certainly improve the basis for extrapolating from high to low doses and from one species to another, they are difficult to acquire and often unavailable.

Regulators are interested in doses to which humans might be exposed, and such doses usually are much lower than those administered in animal studies. Therefore, dose-response assessment often requires extrapolating an expected response curve over a wide range of doses from one or two actual data points. In addition, differences in size and metabolic rates between man and laboratory animals require that doses used experimentally be converted to reflect these differences.

Low-Dose Extrapolation

One may extrapolate to low doses by fitting a mathematical model to animal dose-response data and using the model to predict risks at lower doses corresponding to those experienced by humans. At present, the true shape of the dose-response curve at doses several orders of magnitude below the observation range cannot be determined experimentally. Even the largest study on record-- the ED_{01} study involving 24,000 animals--was designed only to measure the dose corresponding to a 1% increase in tumor incidence. However, regulatory agencies are often concerned about much lower risks (1 in 100,000 to 1 in 1,000). Several methods have been developed to extrapolate from high doses to low doses that would correspond to risk of such magnitudes. A difficulty with low-dose extrapolation is that a number of the extrapolation methods fit the data from animal experiments reasonably well, and it is impossible to distinguish their validity on the basis of goodness of fit. (From a mathematical point of view, distinguishing among these models on the basis of their fit with experimental data would require an extremely large experiment; from a practical point of view, it is probably impossible). As Figure I-2 shows, the dose-response curves derived with different models to diverge below the experimental doses and may diverge substantially in the dose range of interest to regulators. Thus, low-dose extrapolation must be more than a curve-fitting exercise, and considerations of biological plausibility must be taken into account.

Although the five models shown in Figure I-2 may fit experimental data equally well, they are not equally plausible biologically. Most persons in the field would agree that the supralinear model can be disregarded, because it is very difficult to conceive of a biologic mechanism that would give rise to this type of low-dose response. The threshold model is based on the assumption that, below a particular dose (the "threshold" dose of a given carcinogen) there is no adverse effect. This concept is plausible, but not now confirmable. The ED_{01} study showed an apparent threshold for bladder cancers caused by 2-acetylaminofluorene; when the data were replotted on a scale giving greater resolution (OTA, 1981), the number of bladder tumors consistently increased with dose, even at the lowest doses, and no threshold was detected. Another aspect of the debate over thresholds for inducing carcinogenic effects is the argument that agents that act through genotoxic mechanisms are not likely to have a threshold, whereas agents whose effects are mediated by epigenetic mechanisms are possibly more likely to have a threshold. The latter argument is also currently open to scientific challenge. Finally, apparent thresholds observable in animal bioassays cannot be equated with thresholds for entire populations. Even if a threshold exists for individuals, a single threshold would probably not be applicable to the whole population.

Animal-to-Human Dose Extrapolation
In extrapolating from animals to humans, the doses used in bioassays must be adjusted to allow for differ-

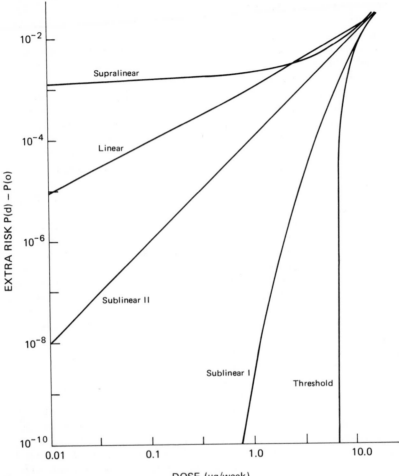

FIGURE I-2 Results of alternative extrapolation models
for the same experimental data. NOTE: Dose-response
functions were developed (Crump, in press) for data from
a benzopyrene carcinogenesis experiment with mice
conducted by Lee and O'Neill (1971).

ences in size and metabolic rates. Several methods currently are used for this adjustment and assume that animal and human risks are equivalent when doses are measured as milligrams per kilogram per day, as milligrams per square meter of body surface area, as parts per million in air, diet, or water, or as milligrams per kilogram per lifetime. Although some methods for conversion are used more frequently than others, a scientific basis for choosing one over the other is not established.

Step 3. Exposure Assessment

The first task of an exposure assessment is the determination of the concentration of the chemical to which humans are exposed. This may be known from direct measurement, but more typically exposure data are incomplete and must be estimated. Models for estimating exposure can be complex, even in the case of structured activity, as occurs in the workplace. Exposure measurements made on a small group (e.g., workers in a particular industrial firm) are often applied to other segments of the worker population.

Exposure assessment in an occupational setting consists primarily of estimation of long-term airborne exposures in the workplace. However, because an agent may be present at various concentrations in diverse occupational settings, a census of exposures is difficult and costly to conduct. In the community environment, the ambient concentrations of chemicals to which people may be exposed can be estimated from emission rates only if the transport and conversion processes are known. Alternative engineering control options require different estimates of the reduction in exposure that may be achieved. For new chemicals with no measurement data at all, rough estimations of exposure are necessary. Some chemical agents are of concern because they are present in foods or may be absorbed when a consumer product is used. Assessments of exposure to such agents are complicated by variations in diet and personal habits among different groups in the population. Even when the amount of an agent in a food can be measured, differences in food storage practices, food preparation, and dietary frequency often lead to a wide variation in the amount of the agent that individuals ingest. Patterns of use affect exposure to many consumer products; for example, a solvent whose vapor is potentially toxic may be used outdoors or it may be used in a small, poorly ventilated room, where the concentration of vapor in the air is much higher.

Another important aspect of exposure assessment is the determination of which groups in the population may be exposed to a chemical agent; some groups may be especially susceptible to adverse health effects. Pregnant women, very young and very old people, and persons with impaired health may be particularly important in exposure assessment. The importance of exposures to a mixture of carcinogens is another factor that needs to be considered in asssssing human exposures. For example, exposure to cigarette smoke and asbestos gives an incidence of cancer that is much greater than anticipated from carcinogenicity data on each substance individually. Because data detecting such synergistic effects are often unavailable, they are often ignored or accounted for by the use of various safety factors.

Step 4. Risk Characterization

Risk characterization, the estimate of the magnitude of the public-health problem, involves no additional scientific knowledge or concepts. However, the exercise of judgment in the aggregation of population groups with varied sensitivity and different exposure may affect the estimate.

SCIENTIFIC AND POLICY JUDGMENTS IN RISK ASSESSMENT

The uncertainties inherent in risk assessment can be grouped in two general categories: missing or ambiguous information on a particular substance and gaps in current scientific theory. When scientific uncertainty is encountered in the risk assessment process, inferential bridges are needed to allow the process to continue. The Committee has defined the points in the risk assessment process where such inferences must be made as components. The judgments made by the scientist/risk assessor for each component of risk assessment often entail a choice among several scientifically plausible options; the Committee has designated these inference options.

COMPONENTS OF RISK ASSESSMENT

A list of components in carcinogenicity risk assessments was compiled by the Committee and is given below. This list is not exhaustive or comprehensive, nor would all components listed be found in every risk assessment. The actual array of components in a particular risk assessment depends on a number of factors, including the types and extent of available data.

Hazard Identification

Epidemiologic Data
* What relative weights should be given to studies with differing results? For example, should positive results outweigh negative results if the studies that yield them are comparable? Should a study be weighted in accord with its statistical power?
* What relative weights should be given to results of different types of epidemiologic studies? For example, should the findings of a prospective study supersede those of a case-control study, or those of a case-control study those of an ecologic study?
* What statistical significance should be required for results to be considered positive?
* Does a study have special characteristics (such as the questionable appropriateness of the control group) that lead one to question the validity of its results?
* What is the significance of a positive finding in a study in which the route of exposure is different from that of a population at potential risk?
* Should evidence on different types of responses be weighted or combined (e.g., data on different tumor sites and data on benign versus malignant tumors)?

Animal-Bioassay Data
* What degree of confirmation of positive results should be necessary? Is a positive result from a single animal study sufficient, or should positive results from two or more animal studies be required? Should negative results be disregarded or given less weight?
* Should a study be weighted according to its quality and statistical power?
* How should evidence of different metabolic pathways or vastly different metabolic rates between animals and humans be factored into a risk assessment?
* How should the occurrence of rare tumors be treated? Should the appearance of rare tumors in a treated group be considered evidence of carcinogenicity even if the finding is not statistically significant?

- How should experimental-animal data be used when the exposure routes in experimental animals and humans are different?
- Should a dose-related increase in tumors be discounted when the tumors in question have high or extremely variable spontaneous rates?
- What statistical significance should be required for results to be considered positive?
- Does an experiment have special characteristics (e.g., the presence of carcinogenic contaminants in the test substance) that lead one to question the validity of its results?
- How should findings of tissue damage or other toxic effects be used in the interpretation of tumor data? Should evidence that tumors may have resulted from these effects be taken to mean that they would not be expected to occur at lower doses?
- Should benign and malignant lesions be counted equally?
- Into what categories should tumors be grouped for statistical purposes?
- Should only increases in the numbers of tumors be considered, or should a decrease in the latent period for tumor occurrence also be used as evidence of carcinogenicity?

Short-Term Test Data
- How much weight should be placed on the results of various short-term tests?
- What degree of confidence do short-term tests add to the results of animal bioassays in the evaluation of carcinogenic risks for humans?
- Should in vitro transformation tests be accorded more weight than bacterial mutagenicity tests in seeking evidence of a possible carcinogenic effect?
- What statistical significance should be required for results to be considered positive?
- How should different results of comparable tests be weighted? Should positive results be accorded greater weight than negative results?

Structural Similarity to Known Carcinogens
- What additional weight does structural similarity add to the results of animal bioassays in the evaluation of carcinogenic risks for humans?

General
* What is the overall weight of the evidence of
carcinogenicity? (This determination must include a
judgment of the quality of the data presented in the
preceding sections.)

Dose-Response Assessment

Epidemiologic Data
* What dose-response models should be used to
extrapolate from observed doses to relevant doses?
* Should dose-response relations be extrapolated
according to best estimates or according to upper confidence limits?
* How should risk estimates be adjusted to account
for a comparatively short follow-up period in an epidemiologic study?
* For what range of health effects should responses
be tabulated? For example, should risk estimates be made
only for specific types of cancer that are unequivocally
related to exposure, or should they apply to all types of
cancers?
* How should exposures to other carcinogens, such
as cigarette smoke, be taken into consideration?
* How should one deal with different temporal exposure patterns in the study population and in the population for which risk estimates are required? For example,
should one assume that lifetime risk is only a function
of total dose, irrespective of whether the dose was
received in early childhood or in old age? Should recent
doses be weighted less than earlier doses?
* How should physiologic characteristics be factored
into the dose-response relation? For example, is there
something about the study group that distinguishes its
response from that of the general population?

Animal-Bioassay Data
* What mathematical models should be used to extrapolate from experimental doses to human exposures?
* Should dose-response relations be extrapolated
according to best estimates or according to upper confidence limits? If the latter, what confidence limits
should be used?
* What factor should be used for interspecies conversion of dose from animals to humans?

   • How should information on comparative metabolic
processes and rates in experimental animals and humans be
used?
   • If data are available on more than one nonhuman
species or genetic strain, how should they be used?
Should only data on the most sensitive species or strain
be used to derive a dose—response function, or should the
data be combined? If data on different species and
strains are to be combined, how should this be accomplished?
   • How should data on different types of tumors in a
single study be combined? Should the assessment be based
on the tumor type that was affected the most (in some
sense) by the exposure? Should data on all tumor types
that exhibit a statistically significant dose—related
increase be used? If so, how? What interpretation
should be given to statistically significant decreases in
tumor incidence at specific sites?

Exposure Assessment*

   • How should one extrapolate exposure measurements
from a small segment of a population to the entire
population?
   • How should one predict dispersion of air pollutants into the atmosphere due to convection, wind cur-
rents, etc., or predict seepage rates of toxic chemicals
into soils and groundwater?
   • How should dietary habits and other variations in
lifestyle, hobbies, and other human activity patterns be
taken into account?
   • Should point estimates or a distribution be used?
   • How should differences in timing, duration, and
age at first exposure be estimated?
   • What is the proper unit of dose?
   • How should one estimate the size and nature of
the populations likely to be exposed?
   • How should exposures of special risk groups, such
as pregnant women and young children, be estimated?

_____

*Current methods and approaches to exposure assessment
appear to be medium— or route—specific. In contrast with
hazard identification and dose—response assessment, exposure assessment has very few components that could be
applicable to all media.

Risk Characterization

* What are the statistical uncertainties in estimating the extent of health effects? How are these
uncertainties to be computed and presented?
* What are the biologic uncertainties in estimating
the extent of health effects? What is their origin? How
will they be estimated? What effect do they have on quantitative estimates? How will the uncertainties be
described to agency decision-makers?
* Which dose-response assessments and exposure
assessments should be used?
* Which population groups should be the primary
targets for protection, and which provide the most
meaningful expression of the health risk?

THE INTERPLAY OF SCIENCE AND POLICY IN RISK ASSESSMENT

A key premise of the proponents of institutional separation of risk assessment is that removal of risk assessment
from the regulatory agencies will result in a clear demar-
cation of the science and policy aspects of regulatory
decision-making. However, policy considerations inevitably affect, and perhaps determine, some of the choices
among the inference options. To examine the types of
judgments required in risk assessment, the Committee has
analyzed several components and the inference options for
each.

Hazard Identification

The Committee has identified 25 components in hazard
identification. These components differ in a number of
ways. However, two major differences germane to the
question considered here are the degree of scientific
uncertainty encountered in each and the effect of
choosing different inference options on the outcome of
the risk assessment. Consider the following examples.

One component of risk assessment is the decision as to
whether to use experimental animal data to infer risks to
humans. Although data from studies of rats and mice may
not always be predictive of adverse health effects in
humans, the scientific validity of this approach is widely
accepted. The use of positive animal data is the more
conservative choice for this component. The use of

negative animal data to determine the absence of carcinogenic risk is less conservative, especially when the sensitivity of the assay is low. (The Committee uses the
term conservative with appropriate modifiers to describe
the degree to which a particular inference option for
components in hazard identification will increase the
likelihood that a substance will be judged to be a
significant hazard to human health).

A component about which there is considerably more
scientific uncertainty than the preceding example is the
question of whether to count all types of benign tumors
as evidence of carcinogenicity. Some benign tumors probably can progress to malignant lesions and some probably
do not. The judgment that benign tumors and malignant
tumors should be counted equally will affect tumor incidence and may influence the yes-no determination in
hazard identification, and it can also affect the dose-
response relation by increasing incidence at the doses
tested. Thus, counting benign tumors is often the more
conservative approach.

The examples just given differ in the degree to which
scientific understanding can inform the judgments to be
made. They are similar, however, in that for each, the
available inference options differ in conservatism. For
many components, this difference in degree of conservatism among plausible inference options is not as clear as
in the preceding examples and depends on the data available on a given substance. For example, the decision to
combine incidences for all tumor types and calculate an
overall tumor incidence can influence the final yes-no
decision in hazard identification. However, in this case,
whether such a choice is more conservative than not combining incidences depends on the incidences for each tumor
type in test and control animals. If the incidence in
control animals is slightly below the incidences in test
animals for all tumor types and individual differences
are not statistically significant, combining all tumor
types would be more conservative. However, if incidences
show no consistent trend and differences are statistically significant for only one tumor type, combining the
tumors would be less conservative.

Dose-Response Assessment

The Committee has identified 13 components of dose-
response assessment. Two major components are high- to
low-dose extrapolation and interspecies dose conversion.

In a recent NRC report on the health effects of
nitrate, nitrite, and N-nitroso compounds (National
Academy of Sciences, 1981), three extrapolation models
(the one-hit model, the multistage model, and the multihit model) were used to estimate the dose of a carcinogenic nitrosamine (dimethylnitrosamine) needed to cause
cancer in one of a million rats. The doses calculated
were 0.03 parts per billion (one-hit), 0.04 ppb (multistage), and 2.7 ppb (multihit); that is, the risk estimate per unit of dose would be lower for the one-hit and
multistage models than for the multihit model for this
experiment.

Other judgments in dose-response assessment that will
affect the final estimate include choice of the experimental data set (from among many that might be available)
to be used to calculate the relation between dose and
incidence of tumors (e.g., use of the most sensitive
animal group will result in the most conservative estimate), choice of a scaling factor for conversion of doses
in animals to humans (the risks calculated can vary by a
factor of up to 35, depending on the method used), and
the decision of whether to combine tumor types in determining incidence (as mentioned earlier, the decision to
lump tumors might be more or less conservative than the
decision not to combine incidences from different tumor
types).

Exposure Assessment

Discussion of specific components in exposure assessment
is complicated by the fact that current methods and
approaches to exposure assessment appear to be medium- or
route-specific. In contrast with hazard identification
and dose-response assessment, exposure assessment has very
few components that could be applicable to all media.
For example, a model describing transport of a chemical
through the atmosphere is necessarily quite different
from a model describing transport through water or soil,
whereas the use of a particular dose-response extrapolation model in dose-response assessment is independent of
the medium or route of exposure. In any event, an
assessor has several options available for estimating
exposure to a particular agent in a particular medium,
and these options will yield more or less conservative
estimates of exposure. Among the options are different
assumptions about the frequency and duration of human

exposure to an agent or medium, rates of intake or con-
tact, and rates of absorption.

Risk Characterization

The final expressions of risk derived in this step will
be used by the regulatory decision-maker when health risks
are weighed against other societal costs and benefits to
determine an appropriate action. Little guidance is
available on how to express uncertainties in the underlying data and on which dose-response assessments and
exposure assessments should be combined to give a final
estimate of possible risk.

Basis for Selecting Inference Options

The Committee has presented some of the more familiar,
and possibly more controversial, components of risk
assessment. A review of the list of components reveals
that many components lack definitive scientific answers,
that the degree of scientific consensus concerning the
best answer varies (some are more controversial among
scientists than others), and that the inference options
available for each component differ in their degree of
conservatism. The choices encountered in risk assessment
rest, to various degrees, on a mixture of scientific fact
and consensus, on informed scientific judgment, and on
policy determinations (the appropriate degree of
conservatism).
    That a scientist makes the choices does not render the
judgments devoid of policy implications. Scientists differ in their opinions of the validity of various options,
even if they are not consciously choosing to be more or
less conservative. In considering whether to use data
from the most sensitive experimental animals for risk
assessment, a scientist may be influenced by the species,
strains, and gender of the animals tested, the characteristics of the tumor, and the conditions of the experiment. A scientist's weighting of these variables may not
easily be expressed explicitly, and the result is a mixture of fact, experience (often called intuition), and
personal values that cannot be disentangled easily. As a
result, the choice made may be perceived by the scientist
as based primarily on informed scientific judgment. From
a regulatory official's point of view, the same choice

may appear to be a value decision as to how conservative
regulatory policy should be, given the lack of a decisive
empirical basis for choice.

A risk assessor, in the absence of a clear indication
based on science, could choose a particular approach
(e.g., the use of an extrapolation model) solely on the
basis of the degree to which it is conservative, i.e., on
the basis of its policy implications. Furthermore, a
desire to err on the side of overprotection of public
health by increasing the estimate of risk could lead an
assessor to choose the most conservative assumptions
throughout the process for components on which science
does not indicate a preferred choice. Such judgments
made in risk assessment are designated risk assessment
policy, that is, policy related to and subservient to the
scientific content of the process, in contrast with policy
invoked to guide risk management decisions, which has
political, social, and economic determinants.

When inference options are chosen primarily on the
basis of policy, risk management considerations (the
desire to regulate or not to regulate) may influence the
choices made by the assessors. The influence can be
generic or ad hoc; i.e., assessments for all chemicals
would consistently use the more or less conservative
inference options, depending on the overall policy orientation of the agency ("generic"), or assessments would
vary from chemical to chemical, with more conservative
options being chosen for substances that the agency wishes
to regulate and less conservative options being chosen for
substances that the agency does not wish to regulate.
(The desire to regulate or not would presumably stem from
substance-specific economic and social considerations.)
The possible influence of risk management considerations,
whether real or perceived, on the policy choices made in
risk assessment has led to reform proposals (reviewed
later in this report) that would separate risk assessment
activities from the regulatory agencies.

Table I-1 recapitulates the terms introduced in this
discussion.

RISK ASSESSMENT IN PRACTICE

This section addresses past agency practices of risk
assessment associated with efforts to regulate toxic
substances.

TABLE I-1 Summary of Terms

Risk Assessment. Risk assessment is the qualitative
or quantitative characterization of the potential health
effects of particular substances on individuals or
populations.

Risk Management. Risk management is the process of
evaluating alternative regulatory options and selecting
among them. A risk assessment may be one of the bases of
risk management.

Steps. Risk assessments comprise many or all of the
following steps: hazard identification, dose-response
assessment, exposure assessment, and risk
characterization.

Components. Steps in risk assessment comprise many
components--points in a risk assessment at which judgments must be made regarding the analytic approach to be
taken.

Inference options. For many components, two or more
inference options are available.

Risk Assessment Policy. Risk assessment policy
consists of the analytic choices that must be made in the
course of a risk assessment. Such choices are based on
both scientific and policy considerations.

RISK ASSESSMENT AND REGULATORY DECISION-MAKING

The regulatory process can be initiated in many ways.
Each regulatory agency typically has jurisdiction over a
large number of substances, but circumstances force an
allocation of resources to a few at a time. The decision
as to which substances to regulate is based, at least in
part, on the degree of hazard. Thus, some notion of relative hazard (implicit or explicit, internally generated
or imposed by outside groups) is necessary. Critics of
federal regulation have contended that the agencies have
not set their priorities sensibly. In general, agency
risk assessments for priority-setting have been more
informal, less systematic, and less visible than those
for establishing regulatory controls.

Agenda-setting involves decisions about which substances should be selected (and often in what order) for more intense formal regulatory review. All programs face this problem, but it assumes different configurations: some programs cover a finite and known set of chemicals that must be reviewed, so the order of the regulatory reviews is the key question, and the primary job of the risk assessor is to help the agency implement a worst-first approach. For example, EPA's pesticides program has long had lists of suspect pesticide ingredients, and agency officials have had to decide which ones warrant formal consideration of cancellation or of new controls. An agency's agenda may also respond to private-sector initiatives (in the case of approval of new drugs or pesticides), conform to statutory directives, or react to new evidence of hazards previously unrecognized or thought to be less serious. This agenda formation phase, too, involves elements of risk assessment by the agency, the Congress, or private-sector entities; that is, there must be some assessment, however informal, that indicates reason for concern.

For many items on an agency's regulatory agenda, hazard identification alone will support a conclusion that a chemical presents little or no risk to human health and should be removed from regulatory consideration, at least until new data warrant renewed concern. If a chemical is found to be potentially dangerous in the hazard-identification step, it could then be taken through the steps of dose-response assessment, exposure assessment, and risk characterization. At any of these steps, the evaluation might indicate that a substance poses little or no risk and therefore can be removed from regulatory consideration until new data indicate a need for reevaluation.

Chemicals that are judged to present appreciable risks to health are candidates for regulatory action, and an agency will begin to develop options for regulating exposures. Regulatory options usually involve specific product or process changes and typically need to be based on extensive engineering and technical knowledge of the affected industry. Evaluation of the regulatory options includes recomputation of the predicted risk, in accord with altered expectations of exposure intensity or numbers of persons exposed.

Many of the activities of regulatory agencies do not conform to this sequential approach. However, regardless of the sequence of steps and the number of steps used to determine whether regulatory action is warranted, risk assessment serves at least two major functions in regulatory decisions: first, it provides an initial assessment of risks, and, if the risk is judged to be important enough to warrant regulatory action, it is used to evaluate the effects of different regulatory options on exposure. In addition, it may be used to set priorities for regulatory consideration and for further toxicity testing.

These varied functions place different requirements on risk assessors, and a single risk assessment method may not be sufficient. A risk assessment to establish testing priorities may appropriately incorporate many worst-case assumptions if there are data gaps, because research should be directed at substances with the most crucial gaps; but such assumptions may be inappropriate for analyzing regulatory controls, particularly if the regulator must ensure that controls do not place undue strains on the economy. In establishing regulatory priorities, the same inference options should be chosen for all chemicals, because the main point of the analysis is to make useful risk comparisons so that agency resources will be used rationally. However, this approach, which may be reasonable for priority-setting, may have to yield to more sophisticated and detailed scientific arguments when a substance's commercial life is at stake and the agency's decision may be challenged in court. Furthermore, the available resources and the resulting analytic care devoted to a risk assessment for deciding regulatory policy are likely to be much greater for analyzing control actions for a single substance than for setting priorities.

THE AGENCIES THAT REGULATE

The approach to risk assessment varies considerably among the four federal agencies. Differences stem primarily from variations in agency structure and differences in statutory mandates and their interpretation.

Organizational Arrangements

The Food and Drug Administration (FDA) is a component of the Department of Health and Human Services, whose Secretary is the formal statutory delegate of the powers exercised by FDA. FDA is headed by a single official, the Commissioner of Food and Drugs, who is appointed by and serves at the pleasure of the Secretary of the Department of Health and Human Services. It is organized in product-related bureaus, each of which employs its own scientists, technicians, compliance officers, and administrators. FDA has a long (75-year) and strong scientific tradition. According to a recent Office of Technology Assessment summary, FDA had taken or proposed action on 24 potential carcinogens by 1981.

Like FDA, the Environmental Protection Agency (EPA) is headed by a single official, but EPA's Administrator is appointed by the President subject to Senate confirmation. Also like FDA, EPA resembles a confederation of relatively discrete programs that are coordinated and overseen by a central management. The agency was established in 1970, but many of its programs (e.g., air and water pollution control and pesticide regulation) predate its formation and previously were housed in and administered by other departments. Other programs, such as those for toxic substances and hazardous waste, are rather new. EPA's research, policy evaluation, and, until recently, enforcement efforts were separated organizationally from the program offices that write regulations. EPA has had the widest experience with regulating carcinogens; as of 1981, it had acted on 56 chemicals in its clean-water program, 29 in its clean-air program, 18 in its pesticide program, and two in its drinking-water program.

The Occupational Safety and Health Administration (OSHA) is part of the Department of Labor. The agency's head is an Assistant Secretary of Labor, who requires Senate confirmation. Although FDA and EPA derive their scientific support largely from their own full-time employees, until the late 1970s OSHA relied on other agencies, primarily the National Institute of Occupational Safety and Health, an agency of the Department of Health and Human Services. This division reflects a conscious congressional choice in 1970 to place the health experts on whom OSHA was expected to rely in an outside environment believed more congenial to scientific inquiry and less vulnerable to political influence. As of 1981, 18 potential carcinogens had been acted on by OSHA.

The Consumer Product Safety Commission (CPSC) enforces five statutes, including the Consumer Product Safety Act and the Federal Hazardous Substances Act. Both empower CPSC to regulate unreasonable risks of injury from products used by consumers in the home, in schools, or in recreation. The much smaller CPSC differs sharply from the other three agencies in two important respects: it does not have a single administrative head, but instead is governed by five Commissioners, who can make major regulatory decisions only by majority vote; and the Commissioners are appointed for fixed terms by the President with Senate confirmation. Before 1981, CPSC had acted on five potential carcinogens.

The four agencies have attempted to coordinate risk assessment activities in the past, most notably through the Interagency Regulatory Liaison Group (IRLG), which formed a work group on risk assessment to develop a guideline for assessing carcinogenic risks. Assisted by scientists from the National Cancer Institute and the National Institute for Environmental Health Sciences, it examined the various approaches used by the four agencies to evaluate evidence of carcinogenicity and to assess risk. The IRLG (1979a,b) then integrated and incorporated these evaluative procedures into a document, "Scientific Bases for Identification of Potential Carcinogens and Estimation of Risks," which described the basis for evaluation of carcinogenic hazards identified through epidemiologic and experimental studies and the methods used for quantitative estimation of carcinogenic risk.

Regulatory Statutes*

Examination of the statutes that the four agencies administer reveals important differences in the standards that govern their decisions. The Office of Technology Assessment has summarized (Table I-2) statutes that pertain to the regulation of carcinogenic chemicals. In particular, the statutes accord different weights to such criteria as risk, costs of control, and technical feasibility. In addition, different modes of regulation vary in their capacity to generate the scientific data necessary to perform comprehensive risk assessments.

Several laws require agencies to balance regulatory costs and benefits. Examples of balancing provisions are found in the Safe Drinking Water Act; the Federal Insecticide, Fungicide, and Rodenticide Act; the Toxic Substances

---

*This discussion draws heavily on the Office of Technology Assessment report, Technologies for Determining Cancer Risks from the Environment, 1981.

Control Act; and the section on fuel additives in the
Clean Air Act. Under such provisions, a risk assessment
can be used to express the nature and extent of public-
health benefits to be attained through regulation.

Some regulatory programs involve the establishment of
technology-based exposure controls. This approach is
followed, for example, in portions of the clean-water
program and the part of the hazardous-wastes program that
deals with waste-incineration standards. In such programs, a risk assessment may be used to show the human
exposure that corresponds to a specific degree of risk or
to calculate the risk remaining after control technologies
are put in place.

Some statutes mandate control techniques to reduce
risks to zero whenever hazard is affirmed. Such techniques include outright bans of products, as envisioned
in the Delaney clause in the Federal Food, Drug, and
Cosmetic Act. In addition, if the concept of a threshold
below which carcinogens pose no risk is not accepted,
strict interpretations of ample margin of safety language
in federal clean-air and clean-water legislation would
require that exposures to carcinogenic pollutants be
reduced to zero. The role of risk assessment in cases
where mandatory control techniques must reduce risks to
zero may be simply to affirm that a hazard exists.

The difference between programs that involve premarketing approval of substances and programs that operate
through post hoc mechanisms, such as environmental emission limits, may have an important influence over the
quality of risk assessments. The most important effect
of this difference may lie in the fact that premarketing
approval programs (such as those for pesticides, for new
human drugs, and for new food additives) empower an agency
to require the submission of sufficient data for a comprehensive risk assessment, whereas other programs tend to
leave agencies to fend for themselves in the acquisition
of necessary data.

There can be little question that differing statutory
standards for decision affect the weight that agencies
accord risk assessments. Like differences in the mode of
regulation, they probably have affected the rigor and
scope of many assessments. If risk is but one of several
criteria that a regulator must consider or if data are
expensive to obtain, it would not be surprising if an
agency devoted less effort to risk assessment. However,
the Committee has not discovered differences in existing
statutes that should impede the adoption of uniform,

TABLE I-2 Public Laws Providing for the Regulation of Exposures to Carcinogens

Legislation (Agency)	Definition of toxics or hazards used for regulation of carcinogens	Degree of protection	Agents regulated as carcinogens (or proposed for regulation)	Basis of the legislation	Remarks
Federal Food, Drug and Cosmetic Act: (FDA)					
Food	Carcinogenicity for *additive* defined by Delaney Clause	No risk permitted, ban of additive	21 food additives and colors	Risk	
	Contaminants	"necessary for the protection of public health..." sec. 406 (346)	Three substances—aflatoxin, PCBs, nitrosamines	Balancing	
Drugs	Carcinogenicity is defined as a risk	Risks and benefits of drug are balanced.	Not determined	Balancing	
Cosmetics	"substance injurious under conditions of use prescribed."	Action taken on the basis that cosmetic is adulterated.	Not determined	Risk. No health claims are allowed for "cosmetics." If claims are made, cosmetic becomes a "drug."	
Occupational Safety and Health Act (OSHA)	Not defined in Act (but OSHA Generic Cancer Policy defines carcinogens on basis of animal test results or epidemiology.)	"adequately assures to the extent feasible that no employee will suffer material impairment of health or functional capacity..." sec. 6(b) (5)	20 substances	Technology (or balancing)	
Clean Air Act (EPA) Sec. 112 (stationary sources)	"an air pollutant... which ...may cause, or contribute to, an increase in mortality or an increase in serious irreversible, or incapacitating reversible, illness." sec. 112(a) (1)	"an ample margin of safety to protect the public health..." sec. 112(b) (1) (B)	Asbestos, beryllium, mercury, vinyl chloride, benzene, radionuclides, and arsenic (an additional 24 substances are being considered)	Risk	Basis of the Airborne Carcinogen Policy

Sec. 202 (vehicles)	"air pollutant from any ...new motor vehicles.... or engine, which...cause, or contribute to, air pollution which may reasonably be anticipated to endanger public health or welfare." sec. 202A(a) (1)	"standards which reflect the greatest degree of emission reduction achieveable through....technology ...available...." sec. 202(b) (3)(a) (1)	Diesel particulates standard	Technology Sec. 202(b) (4) (B) includes a risk-risk test for deciding between pollutant that might result from control attempts.	Sec. 202(b) (4) (A) specifies that no pollution control device, system, or element shall be allowed if it presents an unreasonable risk to health, welfare or safety.
Sec. 211 (fuel additives)	Same as above (211(c) (1)).	Same as above (211(c) (2) (a)).	—	Balancing. Technology-based with consideration of costs, but health-based in requirement that standards provide ample margin of safety.	A cost-benefit comparison of competing control technologies is required.
Clean Water Act (EPA) Sec. 307	Toxic pollutants listed in Committee Report 95-30 of House Committee on Public Works and Transportation. List from consent decree between EDF, NRDC, Citizens for Better Environment and EPA.	Defined by applying BAT economically achieveable (sec. 307(a) (2)), but effluent levels are to "provide(s) an ample margin of safety." (sec. 307(a) (4))	49 substances listed as carcinogens by CAG.	Technology	
Federal Insecticide, Fungicide, and Rodenticide Act and the Federal Environmental Pesticide Control Act (EPA)	One which results in "unreasonable adverse effects on the environment or will involve unreasonable hazard to the survival of a species declared endangered...."	Not specified.	14 rebuttable presumptions against registrations either initiated or completed; nine pesticides voluntarily withdrawn from market.	Sec. 2(bb) Balancing: "unreasonable adverse effects...."	"Unreasonable adverse effects" means "unreasonable risk to man or the environment taking into account the economic, social, and environmental costs and benefits...."

46

TABLE I-2 (Continued)

Legislation (Agency)	Definition of toxics or hazards used for regulation of carcinogens	Degree of protection	Agents regulated as carcinogens (or proposed for regulation)	Basis of the legislation	Remarks
Resource Conservation and Recovery Act (EPA)	One which "may cause, or significantly contribute to an increase in mortality or an increase in serious irreversible, or incapacitating reversible, illness; or, pose a...hazard to human health or the environment...." sec. 1004(5) (A) (B)	"that necessary to protect human health and the environment...." sec. 3002-04	74 substances proposed for listing as hazardous wastes	Risk. The Administrator can order monitoring and set standards for sites.	
Safe Drinking Water Act (EPA)	"contaminant(s) which...may have an adverse effect on the health of persons." sec. 1401(1) (B)	"to the extent feasible...(taking costs into consideration)..." sec. 1412(a) (2)	Trihalomethanes, chemicals formed by reactions between chlorine used as disinfectant and organic chemicals. Two pesticides and 2 metals classified as carcinogens by CAG, but regulated because of other toxicities.	Balancing	
Toxic Substances Control Act (EPA) Sec. 4 (to require testing)	substances which "may present an unreasonable risk of injury to health or the environment." sec. 4(a) (1) (A) (i)	Not specified.	Six chemicals used to make plastics pliable.	Balancing: "unreasonable risk."	
Sec. 6 (to regulate)	substances which "present(s) or will present an unreasonable risk of injury to health or the environment." sec. 6(a)	"to protect adequately against such risk using the least burdensome requirement." sec. 6(a)	PCBs regulated as directed by the law.	Balancing: "unreasonable risk."	

Act	Statutory language		Substances	Criterion	Notes
Sec. 7 (to commence civil action against imminent hazards)	"imminently hazardous chemical substance or mixture means a.... substance or mixture which presents an imminent and unreasonable risk of serious or widespread injury to health or the environment."	Based on degree of protection in sec. 6			
Federal Hazardous Substances Act (CPSC)	"any substance (other than a radioactive substance) which has the capacity to produce personal injury or illness . . ." 15 USC sec.	"establish such reasonable variations or additional label requirements. . . . necessary for the protection of public health and safety. . ." 15 USC sec.		Risk	"Highly toxic" defined as capacity to cause death, thus toxicity may be limited to acute toxicity.
Consumer Product Safety Act (CPSC)	"products which present unreasonable risks of injury. . . in commerce," and ". . "risk of injury" means a risk of death, personal injury or serious or frequent injury." 15 USC sec. 2051 "imminently hazardous consumer product' means consumer product which presents imminent and unreasonable risk of death, serious illness or severe personal injury." 15 USC sec. 2061	"standard shall be reasonably necessary to prevent or reduce an unreasonable risk of injury." 15 USC sec. 2056	Five substances: asbestos, benzene, benzidine (and benzidine-based dyes and pigments), vinyl chloride, "tris"	Balancing: "unreasonable"	Standards are to be expressed, wherever feasible, as performance requirements.

SOURCE: Office of Technology Assessment, Technologies for Determining Cancer Risks from the Environment, 1981.

government-wide risk assessment guidelines. Indeed, it is not satisfied that there are legal bases for inter-agency differences in the performance--as distinct from the use--of risk assessment for chronic health hazards.

CONCLUSIONS

On the basis of a review of the nature and the policy context of risk assessment, the Committee has drawn the following general conclusions:

1. _Risk assessment is only one aspect of the process of regulatory control of hazardous substances. Therefore, improvements in risk assessment methods cannot be assumed to eliminate controversy over federal risk management decisions._

Restrictive regulation has seemed onerous to manufac-turers, distributors, and users of products judged useful and valuable; conversely, inaction and delay with respect to regulatory proceedings have appeared callous and irresponsible to others. These dissatisfactions have been manifested in many ways, including criticism of risk assessment processes. The Committee believes that much of this criticism is inappropriately directed and gives rise to an unrealistic expectation that modifying risk assessment procedures will result in regulatory decisions more acceptable to the critics. Certainly risk assessment can and should be improved, with salutary effects on the appropriateness of regulatory decisions. However, risk management, although it uses risk assessment, is driven by political, social, and economic forces, and regulatory decisions will continue to arouse controversy and conflict.

2. _Risk assessment is an analytic process that is firmly based on scientific considerations, but it also requires judgments to be made when the available informa-tion is incomplete. These judgments inevitably draw on both scientific and policy considerations._

The primary problem with risk assessment is that the information on which decisions must be based is usually inadequate. Because the decisions cannot wait, the gaps in information must be bridged by inference and belief, and these cannot be evaluated in the same way as facts. Improving the quality and comprehensiveness of knowledge is by far the most effective way to improve risk assessment, but some limitations are inherent and unresolvable, and inferences will always be required. Although we conclude that the mixing of science and policy in risk assessment cannot be eliminated, we believe that most of the intrusions of policy can be identified and that a major contribution to the integrity of the risk assessment process would be the development of a procedure to ensure that the judgments made in risk assessments, and the underlying rationale for such judgments, are made explicit.

3. <u>Two kinds of policy can potentially affect risk assessment: that which is inherent in the assessment process itself and that which governs the selection of regulatory options. The latter, risk management policy, should not be allowed to control the former, risk assessment policy.</u>
Risk management policy, by its very nature, must entail value judgments related to public perceptions of risk and to information on risks, benefits, and costs of control strategies for each substance considered for regulation. Such information varies from substance to substance, so the judgments made in risk management must be case-specific. If such case-specific considerations as a substance's economic importance, which are appropriate to risk management, influence the judgments made in the risk assessment process, the integrity of the risk assessment process will be seriously undermined. Even the <u>perception</u> that risk management considerations are influencing the conduct of risk assessment in an important way will cause the assessment and regulatory decisions based on them to lack credibility.

4. <u>Risk assessment suffers from the current absence of a mechanism for addressing generic issues in isolation from specific risk management decisions.</u>
Although the practice of risk assessment has progressed in recent years, there is currently no mechanism for stimulating and monitoring advances on generic questions in relevant scientific fields or for the timely dissemination of such information to risk assessors.

REFERENCES

Crump, K. S. In press. Issues related to carcinogenic risk assessment from animal bioassay data. Paper

presented May 1981 at the International School of
Technological Risk Assessment, a NATO Advanced Study
Institute, Erice, Italy.

IRLG (Interagency Regulatory Liaison Group), Work Group
on Risk Assessment. 1979a. Scientific bases for
identification of potential carcinogens and estimation
of risks. Fed. Reg. 44:39858.

IRLG (Interagency Regulatory Liaison Group), Work Group
on Risk Assessment. 1979b. Scientific bases for
identification of potential carcinogens and estimation
of risks. J. Natl. Cancer Inst. 63:242.

Lee, P. N., and J. A. O'Neill. 1971. The effect both of
time and dose applied on tumor incidence rate in
benzopyrene skin painting experiments. Brit. J.
Cancer 25:759-770.

National Academy of Sciences. 1981. The Health Effects
of Nitrate, Nitrite, and N-Nitroso Compounds.
Washington, D.C.: National Academy Press. 544 pp.

OTA (Office of Technology Assessment). 1981. Assessment
of the Technologies for Determining Cancer Risks from
the Environment. 240 pp.

II
Inference Guidelines for Risk Assessment

INTRODUCTION AND DEFINITIONS

An <u>inference guideline</u>* is an explicit statement of a
predetermined choice among the options that arise in
inferring human risk from data that are not fully adequate or not drawn directly from human experience. A
guideline might, for example, specify the mathematical
model to be used to estimate the effects of exposure at
low doses from observations based on higher doses. The
most important feature of guideline use is that it changes
the risk assessment process from one in which inference
options are selected on a substance-by-substance basis to
one in which they are selected once and thereafter

---

*The Committee hopes to avoid any misunderstanding result-
ing from its use of the terms <u>inference guideline</u> and
<u>guideline</u> (used for brevity in lieu of <u>inference guide-</u>
<u>line</u>). This terminology is potentially confusing, because
<u>guidelines</u> can be understood as codified principles ad-
dressed to a particular subject matter, risk assessment,
or as describing the legal weight of any codified standards or principles. For the Committee, it has the former
meaning. Inference guidelines are the principles followed
by risk assessors in interpreting and reaching judgments
based on scientific data. (Thus, our inference guidelines are distinct from the standards for toxicologic and
other testing standards that many regulatory agencies and
scientific bodies have adopted to govern, or at least
influence, the generation of data later used in risk
assessment.)

For many lawyers, the term <u>guideline</u> connotes the
weight to be given to any set of codified principles, not

applied to an entire series of chemicals. In the absence
of guidelines, assessors may well select the same inference options for substance after substance in a given
agency program, and a common set of inference options may
emerge, in common law fashion, from their consistent
application in the program. But even the continued use
of the same set of inference options over time does not
necessarily imply that the assessors would make the same
choices for every substance. Furthermore, outsiders
would have no way of knowing what the common set is. In
contrast, the use of guidelines makes more evident the
generic choice of inference options, which we have seen
in Chapter I, is based on both scientific and risk
assessment policy considerations.

HISTORY OF THE USE OF GUIDELINES

SAFETY EVALUATION GUIDELINES FOR EFFECTS OTHER THAN CANCER

The development and use of guidelines by a regulatory
agency first became of major importance after Congress

---

only those addressed to risk assessment, in legal proceedings. The Food and Drug Administration, for example,
has defined a guideline as an official pronouncement of
the agency describing a procedure that satisfies legal
requirements, but is not mandated by law. A more complete
treatment of the distinction between binding regulations
and other formal agency pronouncements appears in the
section of this chapter entitled "Degree to Which Guidelines May Be Binding on an Agency and a Regulated Party."
   The Committee has used the term guideline to describe
the principles by which risk assessments are to be performed, because that is the term Congress used in the
legislation that authorized this study. The Committee
was asked to consider the feasibility of establishing
uniform "risk assessment guidelines." There is no evidence that Congress was aware of the different meanings
of the term. It obviously was seeking advice about the
intellectual and scientific bases for codified principles
for risk assessment, not the appropriate legal form for
their adoption. Faced with possible confusion no matter
which terminology it chose, the Committee has retained
the language that Congress itself used to describe our
inquiry.

enacted amendments to the Federal Food, Drug, and Cosmetics Act in the 1950s and early 1960s. These laws, as applied to noncarcinogenic agents, required that food additives, color additives, drugs for animals, and pesticides be shown to be safe under their intended conditions of use before premarket approval by the Food and Drug Administration (FDA). The agency developed guidelines to provide a systematic way to deal with the legal requirements embodied in the amendments. Although guidelines for the conduct of various types of toxicity tests received greatest notice, some attention was given to the problem of data interpretation for inferring human risk. For example, a 1959 publication written by several members of the FDA Division of Pharmacology, Appraisal of the Safety of Chemicals in Foods, Drugs, and Cosmetics, is devoted primarily to toxicity testing methods, but contains one chapter called "Some Interpretative Problems in Evaluating the Safety of Food Additives" (Lehman et al., 1959). Although that publication, which served as a guide for both FDA and the regulated industry for at least a decade, was never published as a regulation, it was widely accepted by affected industrial concerns.

In all cases except that of carcinogens, establishment of acceptable intakes was accomplished by applying safety factors to experimentally derived no-observed-effect exposures. Testing involved mostly the use of acute and subchronic (90-day) animal tests, although some long-term tests were required. The use of safety factors to establish acceptable intakes was also recommended by the Food Protection Committee of the National Research Council (NRC/NAS, 1970) and adopted by the Joint Food and Agricultural Organization and World Health Organization Expert Committees on Food Additives (1972) and Pesticide Residues (1965). This approach continues to be used for noncarcinogenic food additives and pesticides and, in slightly modified form, to define acceptable exposures to occupational and various environmental pollutants.

These methods of assigning acceptable limits of exposure imply that the application of safety factors of various magnitudes to experimentally derived no-observed-effect exposures will ensure low risk. The acceptable exposure, whether expressed as an acceptable daily intake for a food additive or as a permissible exposure limit for an occupational agent, is derived by imposing untested assumptions (e.g., about the likely nature of dose-response relations at low doses) and by drawing inferences from sparse data. Safety evaluation schemes may therefore

be classified as a set of guidelines that emphasize testing methods heavily and that afford methods of inference
only scant attention.

Recent efforts have dealt more directly with developing
guidelines for risk assessment of noncarcinogenic effects.
The Environmental Protection Agency (EPA) has proposed
guidelines for chemical mutagenesis (EPA, 1980a) and has
collected public comments on them, but has yet to publish
a final rule. In addition, the agency cosponsored two
conferences with Oak Ridge National Laboratory on risk
assessment methods for reproductive and teratogenic
effects; the proceedings of the conferences have been
published (ORNL/EPA, 1982). The Interagency Regulatory
Liaison Group began to develop guidelines for risk
assessment of reproductive and teratogenic effects, but
the effort ceased with the disbanding of the group in
1981. The March of Dimes Birth Defects Foundation (1981)
has published the proceedings of a conference dealing
with guidelines for studies of human populations exposed
to mutagenic and reproductive hazards. Despite the
increasing interest in noncarcinogenic effects, methods
of estimating the risk of these effects have not been the
subject of major public and scientific debate; attention
has been devoted mainly to carcinogenic risk assessment.
Much more critical review of the inferential methods for
assigning risks to noncarcinogenic agents is warranted.

GUIDELINES FOR CARCINOGENIC RISK

Until the late 1950s, few agents, either chemical or
physical, had been regulated in this country on the basis
of their carcinogenic action. One important regulated
agent was ionizing radiation. Permissible exposures to
radiation were set in a manner similar to that for noncarcinogenic agents, by application of safety factors applied
to specified exposures. In the debate over health effects
of radioactive fallout from atomic weapons tests in the
1950s, evidence to support a nonthreshold theory for
cancer induction emerged. Evidence was also accumulated
to indicate that the nonthreshold theory might be applicable to chemical carcinogens. It was in this context
that Congress enacted statutes* in the 1950s and early

---

*The enactment of these statutes did not necessarily
bring a unique new concept to FDA. In the early 1950s,

1960s that required FDA to ban the use of food and color additives shown to be carcinogenic. The assumption, which differed from that underlying safety evaluation of noncarcinogens, was that no exposure could be presumed safe. Thus, a full risk assessment scheme was not needed for carcinogens. The process stopped at hazard identification.

Many factors contributed to the later use of dose-response assessment, exposure assessment, and risk characterization to determine quantitative estimates of risk. One of these may have been the growing perception during the 1960s and 1970s that many kinds of risk could not be eliminated completely without unacceptable social and economic consequences. New laws reflecting this belief were enacted, and some agencies were required to balance the risk posed by carcinogenic agents against their perceived benefits. Quantitative risk assessment was the system developed to estimate the risk side of the balance. Over a period of 2 decades, various expert committees sponsored by government agencies and other organizations published numerous reports dealing with carcinogenicity evaluation. Most of these were state-of-the art reports on aspects of carcinogenicity inference, and many suggested guidelines for hazard identification. More recent reports have dealt explicitly with quantitative risk assessment. The impetus for producing these reports was probably a belief in the federal research and regulatory communities that some scientific principles related to carcinogenicity data evaluation had to be continually reexamined and reaffirmed. This belief pervaded the public-health establishment not only in the United States, but also in other countries and in the United Nations.

The following discussion examines efforts to develop and apply guidelines for the evaluation of carcinogenicity data by the federal regulatory agencies and the International Agency for Research on Cancer over the last decade--efforts that developed out of 2 decades of scientific consensus-building.

---

before their enactment, the agency had prohibited three food additives on the grounds that they were found to be carcinogenic in test animals.

International Agency for Research on Cancer (IARC)

In 1971, the International Agency for Research on Cancer
(IARC), an agency of the World Health Organization, began
publication of a series of monographs on known and suspected carcinogens. These monographs are prepared by
international groups of experts assembled by IARC, who
critically review pertinent literature and draw conclusions regarding the carcinogenicity of various substances.
The results of IARC reviews and evaluations are widely
accepted. The guidelines used for evaluation by the IARC
expert committees are set forth in the monographs. They
are expressed in very general terms and are related to
only six components of hazard identification, completely
covered in six pages of text. A major feature of the
guidelines is the presentation of criteria that classify
the evidence of suspected carcinogens as sufficient or
limited. The IARC allows the expert committees considerable latitude to evaluate many inference options on a
case-by-case basis, although the agency appears to insist
on adherence to the few stated guidelines.

Food and Drug Administration

The 1958 Food Additives Amendment to the Food, Drug, and
Cosmetics Act prohibited the use of food additives found
to be carcinogenic. The law was also interpreted as
prohibiting FDA approval of any drug, for use in animals
produced for human food, that had been shown to cause
cancer. In 1962, by congressional amendment, FDA was
permitted to approve the use of a carcinogenic animal
drug if the agency was convinced that no residue of a
drug would be found in edible tissues of the treated
animals. Congress specified that FDA was to prescribe
the analytic methods for verifying the absence of
residues. This directive proved to be unworkable, for
two reasons: progress in analytic chemistry was so rapid
that approved methods of analysis quickly became obsolete
and improved detection methods showed that no drug administered to animals is ever entirely absent from animal
tissues. The problem of enforcing the 1962 amendment was
highlighted in the early 1970s, when diethylstilbestrol
residues were discovered in beef liver with highly sensitive, but as yet unapproved, analytic methods.

In an attempt to provide a consistent and predictable
procedure for approving methods to search for drug resi-

dues, FDA proposed sensitivity-of-method guidelines in
the form of regulations (FDA, 1973, 1977, 1979b). Rather
than gear criteria to an analytic technique, the agency
defined its standards in terms of risk. It proposed that
any assay approved for controlling a carcinogenic drug
must be capable of measuring residues that present more
than an insignificant risk of cancer, and specified a
10^{-6} lifetime risk of cancer as a quantitative criterion of insignificance. If a drug sponsor could provide a
detection method capable of measuring residues posing a
risk of this magnitude or greater, FDA would ignore residues that could not be detected with this method. Thus,
FDA found guidelines for quantitative estimation of risk
necessary. FDA's sensitivity-of-method guidelines are
unique in several ways. They address a narrow though
complex set of issues encountered in regulating a single
class of products, animal drugs. Although they deal to a
large extent with testing, they were the first to address
quantitative risk assessment methods, listing assumptions
for dose–response assessment, exposure assessment, and
risk characterization. And they are the only guidelines
that attempt to establish a definition of significant
risk. The guidelines have yet to be adopted, a decade
after they were first proposed, but the agency has applied
the methods of quantitative risk assessment embodied in
the sensitivity-of-method document in connection with the
regulation not only of animal drugs, but also of food
contaminants, such as aflatoxin (FDA, 1979a) and trace
constituents of some additives (FDA, 1982b). The
sensitivity-of-method guidelines were proposed as regulations, as were the cancer guidelines of the Occupational
Safety and Health Administration (OSHA). In both cases,
regulation engendered substantial controversy. The major
debate over the sensitivity-of-method guidelines has dealt
not so much with risk assessment or the definition of
significant risk as with the amount and cost of testing
that FDA would require from industry before product
approval.

Environmental Protection Agency

During the early to middle 1970s, EPA initiated actions
to prohibit or restrict the use of several pesticides.
The agency lacked internal procedures for assessing
carcinogenic risk and relied heavily on the judgment of
scientists outside EPA. Attorneys for EPA, in summar-

izing the testimony of their expert witnesses during
administrative hearings on actions against the pesticides, set forth several statements that, in the legal
brief, were referred to as cancer principles (EPA, 1972,
1975). They conveyed the idea that the only acceptable
degree of regulation would be a total ban on exposures.
The principles, perceived as EPA's cancer policy, incurred
wide criticism from the scientific community, the private
sector, and Congress. The impracticability of achieving
zero risk on a broad scale for a large number of economi-
cally important chemicals became increasingly apparent.
In response to this new perception, and perhaps out of a
desire to avoid misunderstanding of its cancer policy,
the EPA became the first agency to adopt formal guidelines
embracing a two-step process of risk assessment (EPA,
1976). The first step is a determination of whether a
particular substance constitutes a cancer risk (hazard
identification). The second step is a determination of
what regulatory action, if any, should be taken to reduce
the risk. As part of the second step, the agency explicitly endorses the use of quantitative risk assessment as
the means of determining the magnitude of the likely
impact of a potential human carcinogen on public health.
These guidelines were not published as regulations and
enjoy fairly wide acceptance from most interested parties. As stated in the preface to the guidelines, they
were published to improve agency procedures, to provide
public notice of the approach that EPA would take, and to
stimulate commentary from all sources on that approach.
The guidelines were probably more important as a statement of a novel approach to risk assessment than for their
content. They are quite general, cover less than a page
of Federal Register text, and address only a few components of hazard identification, dose-response assessment,
exposure assessment, and risk characterization. More
detailed guidelines that specify assumptions for the
choice of extrapolation models, scaling factors, and
other elements of dose-response assessment were published
in 1980 by program offices in EPA (EPA, 1980b). These
rely in part on the Interagency Regulatory Liaison Group
(IRLG) guidelines (IRLG, 1979a) and are currently
undergoing review.

Occupational Safety and Health Administration

In 1977, OSHA published guidelines in a proposed regulation, "Identification, Classification, and Regulation of

Toxic Substances Posing a Potential Occupational Risk of Cancer" (OSHA, 1977); after extensive administrative hearings, it published a final rule in 1980 (OSHA, 1980). The guidelines proved to be highly controversial, and the hearings were marked by vigorous debate on almost every component of risk assessment covered by the guidelines.

The OSHA rule, written by agency staff, was a detailed scientific and regulatory document that took several hundred pages of Federal Register text and addressed almost every component of hazard identification. The final rule did not address exposure assessment and rejected the use of dose-response assessment for any regulatory purpose except priority-setting. The main purposes of the guidelines, as stated in the preface, were to streamline the process of risk assessment, to speed up regulation, and to reduce the workload of agency staff. Another purpose was to foster continuity of approach, even in the face of changes of policy-makers. OSHA staff perceived that the case-by-case approach to risk assessment was long and time-consuming, because the same controversial questions had to be argued each time a chemical was under consideration for regulation. The agency believed that the generic approach to risk assessment would reduce debate on these questions; the controversial issues could be decided once, incorporated into guidelines, and applied to all chemicals. For reasons of efficiency, the guidelines were written in language that permitted little deviation from the judgments embodied in them. Because they were written as regulations, regulated parties were required to abide by them. The agency has not used the rule as a basis for any published scientific assessment of carcinogenic hazard. It was revised in 1981 (OSHA, 1981) to accommodate the Supreme Court's ruling on benzene, which required that OSHA make a finding that the risk to workers in the absence of regulation was significant and would be reduced by the proposed standard. But this change and additional amendments were recently withdrawn, and the entire policy is under reconsideration (OSHA, 1982).

Consumer Product Safety Commission

The Consumer Product Safety Commission (CPSC) proposed cancer guidelines dealing mainly with hazard identification (CPSC, 1978). Ten components related to that step were addressed in several pages of Federal Register text.

Some minor attention was given to exposure assessment and dose-response assessment, for priority-setting purposes only. The rationale for publishing the guidelines, as stated in the preface of that document, was to establish CPSC's general principles and to solicit comments on them, to assist the general public and the regulated industries in understanding standards that CPSC would apply and regulatory actions that it was likely to take, and to set forth its approach to some issues that tended to recur in each case. The guidelines had no regulatory status; they were a statement of selected inference options to which the agency would adhere. The CPSC guidelines were never used; they were challenged in court, and the court ruled that CPSC had promulgated them illegally inasmuch as they were adopted without an opportunity for public comment. Furthermore, at that time CPSC had decided to rely on the guidelines of IRLG.

Interagency Regulatory Liaison Group

The four agencies represented in IRLG undertook the task of developing guidelines to "ensure that the regulatory agencies evaluate carcinogenic risk consistently." In 1979, after an 18-month interagency effort, IRLG published a report, "Scientific Bases for Identification of Potential Carcinogens and Estimation of Risk." The report was prepared by personnel of CPSC, EPA, FDA, and OSHA, with the assistance of senior scientists from the National Cancer Institute and the National Institute of Environmental Health Sciences. It was published in a scientific journal (IRLG, 1979b) and in the Federal Register (IRLG, 1979a); IRLG requested public comment in the Federal Register. The IRLG report was said to represent an interagency consensus on the scientific aspects of carcinogenic risk assessment.* It was the most comprehensive set of guidelines that had been developed for agency use, addressing most components of hazard identification and dose-response assessment with some general discussion of

---

*Because rule-making was under way in connection with its cancer policy, OSHA declined to participate in the IRLG notice and comment procedure. After the report was completed, the Food Safety Quality Service of the U.S. Department of Agriculture joined IRLG and participated in the notice and comment.

exposure assessment and risk characterization; it had, however, no official legal status. The report was note-worthy, in that it constituted the first evidence that all the federal regulatory agencies agreed on the infer-ence options applicable to the identification of carcin-ogenic hazards and measurement of risks. The document made clear, however, that not all the agencies were bound to conduct quantitative assessments; it stated only that, if such assessments were to be conducted, they would be conducted uniformly. This language was probably a con-cession to OSHA's view, as expressed in its cancer policy, that quantitative risk assessment was to play no more than a priority-setting role in that agency's regulatory activities. Almost immediately after its publication, the IRLG report was adopted by the President's Regulatory Council and incorporated as the scientific basis of the Council's government-wide statement on regulation of chemical carcinogens. The Council viewed the IRLG guide-lines as a major step in reducing inconsistency, dupli-cation of effort, and lack of coordination among agencies in carcinogenic risk assessment (Regulatory Council, 1979).

The scientific aspects of the final OSHA cancer policy, which was written to allow less latitude in the choice of inference options, were, nevertheless, in general agree-ment with the IRLG guidelines. CPSC and EPA stated that they relied on the IRLG document, but the degree to which they rely on it today is not clear. FDA has made no statement other than that associated with the document's initial publication; in fact, in a recent proposal con-cerning the application of risk assessment to a class of trace constituents of additives, FDA did not even cite the IRLG document as a reference (FDA, 1982b). Although IRLG received a great deal of public comment on the guide-lines, no report of the agencies' review of these comments has appeared. In fact, the document was heavily criti-cized by industry, because it was published in its final form and adopted before the comments could be analyzed and revisions incorporated. The Reagan Administration has officially disbanded the entire IRLG effort, so it is unlikely that review of the public comments will ever occur.

Although the IRLG charter was not renewed, a similar group has been established, but one that is coordinated by the White House Office of Science and Technology Policy. This group has prepared a draft document on the scientific basis of risk assessment and has distributed

it for comment (OSTP, 1982). The group anticipates that
this document may serve as a reference point for later
development of general guidelines for the agencies.

VARIATION IN THE FORM OF GUIDELINES

COMPREHENSIVENESS

Guidelines developed by agencies in the past have varied
in the extent to which they have addressed each of the
steps of risk assessment. IARC's guidelines address only
hazard identification; OSHA's guidelines (1980) dealt
mainly with hazard identification, with some discussion
of dose-response assessment and none of exposure assessment and risk characterization; and IRLG's guidelines
focused in detail on hazard identification and dose-
response assessment, with some discussion of exposure
assessment and risk characterization.

Guidelines also have varied in the extent to which
they have addressed the components of the risk assessment
steps. IARC's guidelines address a small number of
components. Study of the latest IARC monograph (1982)
reveals only six selected options that deal with inference
of risk: treatment of benign versus malignant tumors, the
choice of statistical methods for application of data from
animal studies, the relevance of negative results of epidemiologic studies, the evaluation of tumors that occur
spontaneously, the utility of short-term tests, and the
overall weighting of evidence. The OSHA (1980) and IRLG
documents, in contrast, each discussed and embraced over
20 selected options dealing with hazard identification.

EXTENT OF DETAIL

Guidelines have differed not only in their comprehensiveness, but also in the detail with which they have treated
specific components of risk assessment. When the content
of a guideline is detailed, the assessor is presented with
more complete information than would be available from a
more general guideline. For example, the statement in
IARC's guidelines on benign tumors is general, compared
with that in the IRLG guidelines. IARC concludes briefly:

   If a substance is found to induce only benign
   tumours in experimental animals, it should be

suspected of being a carcinogen and requires
further investigation.

The IRLG document made a similar statement, but in
addition elaborated on several issues relevant to the
evaluation of benign tumors that are not mentioned by
IARC--e.g., evaluation of tumor incidence when both benign
and malignant tumors are present; a listing of tumor types
commonly observed as benign in test animals, but known to
progress to frank malignant stages; evaluation of the
quality of a histologic examination that might be presented as evidence; and an illustrative example of the
dependence of response on the genetic characteristics of
the test animal. The additional material could have been
used by an assessor, particularly one not familiar with
the newest information on benign tumors, to ensure that a
more thorough analysis of the relevant issues had been
performed.

FLEXIBILITY

Detail can often be confused with inflexibility, and it
is important to make a distinction between these characteristics. Certainly, detailed guidelines can be inflexible if the detail is designed to limit agency discretion,
and thus public debate, on an issue that is subject to
multiple scientific interpretations. However, detailed
guidelines can have quite a different effect if their
intent is to provide an assessor with background information that describes the complexity of an issue, with
nuances that may influence particular judgments, or with
examples of cases that are legitimate exceptions to the
general rule.
    As described in Chapter I, almost all components of
risk assessment theoretically embrace one or more inference options. For example, in determining which dose-
response curve to choose, the biologically plausible
inference options may include the linear, multistage,
sublinear, and threshold models. A guideline usually
prefers one option, although some guidelines permit the
selection of more than one or of all the options. The
preferred inference option may be viewed as a default
option, i.e., the option chosen on the basis of risk
assessment policy that appears to be the best choice in
the absence of data to the contrary. A guideline may be
said to be flexible according to the degree to which it

allows the default option to be superseded by another
inference option as a result of convincing scientific
evidence.*

Comparison of IRLG's guidelines with OSHA's guidelines
illustrates how comprehensive and detailed guidelines
have varied in flexibility. On the issue of benign versus
malignant tumors, IRLG's guideline stated:

> The induction of benign neoplasms would, therefore,
> be considered evidence of carcinogenic activity
> unless definitive evidence is provided that the
> test chemical is incapable of inducing malignant
> neoplasms.

The guideline did not attempt to define the type of definitive evidence that would be needed to demonstrate that a
"test chemical is incapable of inducing malignant neo-
plasms." In contrast, OSHA created strict minimal
criteria for acceptance of such evidence:

> (i) Benign tumors. Results based on the induc-
> tion of benign or malignant tumors, or both, will
> be used to establish a qualitative inference of
> carcinogenic hazard to workers. Arguments that
> substances that induce benign tumors do not
> present a carcinogenic risk to workers will be
> considered only if evidence that meets the
> criteria set forth in 1990.144(e) is provided.

Section 1990.144(e) stated:

> (e) Benign tumors. The Secretary will consider
> evidence that the substance subject to the rule-
> making proceeding is capable only of inducing
> benign tumors in human or experimental animals
> provided that the evidence for the specific
> substance meets the following criteria:
> Criteria. (i) Data are available from at least
> two well-conducted bioassays in each of two species
> of mammals (or from equivalent evidence in more
> than two species).

---

*Flexibility is also intimately related to the legal
weight that the agency desires a guideline to have; the
implications for flexibility of adopting guidelines under
different legal authorities are reviewed in the next
section.

(ii) Each of the bioassays to be considered has
been conducted for the full lifetime of the
experimental animals.

(iii) The relevant tissue slides are made available to OSHA or its designee and the diagnoses of
the tumors as benign are made by at least one
qualified pathologist who has personally examined
each of the slides and who provides specific
diagnostic criteria and descriptions; and

(iv) All of the induced tumors must be shown to
belong to a type which is known not to progress to
malignancy or to be at a benign stage when
observed. In the latter case, data must be
presented to show that multiple sections of the
affected organ(s) were adequately examined to
search for invasion of the tumor cells into
adjacent tissue, and that multiple sections of
other organs were adequately examined to search
for tumor metastases.

By leaving open the type of evidence needed to supersede the default option (benign tumors should be considered evidence of carcinogenic activity), IRLG allowed
more flexibility than OSHA.

In no case did the IRLG guidelines attempt to restrict
the type of evidence that would be needed for acceptance
of alternative interpretations. In contrast, OSHA specified minimal criteria for acceptance of alternative
interpretations on the issues of negative epidemiologic
studies, proof of metabolic differences between animals
and humans, and rejection of the use of data from testing
at high doses. By invoking such criteria, OSHA attempted
to limit the definition of acceptable interpretation and,
in so doing, eliminate or reduce scientific debate on
controversial issues in its rule-making proceedings.

IRLG also created flexibility by not choosing a default
option, i.e., by citing a range of possible inference
options to be used in a risk assessment. The statement
on interspecies conversion factors illustrates this point:

Several species-conversion factors should be considered in estimating risk levels for humans from
data obtained in another species.

All OSHA guidelines were restricted to the choice of a
single inference option.

DEGREE TO WHICH GUIDELINES MAY BE BINDING
ON AN AGENCY AND A REGULATED PARTY

The guidelines developed by or for regulatory agencies may
vary in their legal status and thus in their procedural
implications. For example, OSHA's guidelines (1980)
appeared as regulations formally published, after opportunity for public comment, in the Federal Register. In
contrast, EPA's guidelines (1976), although eventually
printed in the Federal Register, have never been officially subjected to public comment and do not purport to be
regulations.

To appreciate the practical differences among the
approaches that an agency might follow, it is useful to
distinguish three types of administrative documents:
regulations (or, synonymously, rules), established procedures (a term we have devised to refer to agency pronouncements that are in some contexts referred to as
guidelines), and recommendations. There is no single
authoritative definition of the latter two types of
document. The discussion here is an attempt to reflect
common understanding; it draws as well on the practice,
but not the terminology of one agency, FDA (1982a).* An
illustration will illuminate the practical differences
among these three types of documents. Suppose that an
agency decides to adopt, as one of its risk assessment
guidelines, the default option that benign tumors should
be aggregated with malignant tumors in determining whether
a mammalian bioassay demonstrates that an agent causes
cancer in the test species. This guideline could be
adopted as a regulation, as what we term an established
procedure, or simply as a recommendation. For internal
purposes, it is not likely to matter which form the

---

*FDA officially recognizes three types of documents:
binding regulations, guidelines, and recommendations.
That terminology is potentially confusing here, because
we have given guidelines a special meaning, connoting
codified principles for risk assessment, that diverges
from FDA's legal definition. The reader is referred to
the footnote at the beginning of this chapter for a more
complete treatment of this discrepancy. We have therefore coined the substitute phrase established procedures,
to describe any standards of criteria for fulfilling a
regulatory requirement that the agency commits itself to
follow until they are formally revoked or revised.

agency's guideline takes. If the guideline is understood
to represent prevailing agency policy, the agency's managers can assume that assessors will adhere to it in evaluating test data, regardless of its form. Important
differences will be observed, however, in the guideline's
impact on interested third parties.

If the guideline were adopted as a regulation, it would
be reciprocally binding. Neither the agency nor any private party would be free to argue in a regulatory proceeding that benign and malignant tumors should never be
aggregated or should not in a particular instance be
aggregated; the agency's regulation would render such
arguments legally irrelevant. It is precisely this effect
of regulations--i.e., their treatment of previously con-
tested (and in theory still contestable) issues as author-
itatively resolved--that OSHA sought when it published
its risk assessment guidelines as regulations.

If the guidelines were merely a recommendation, manufacturers of chemicals under evaluation would not be bound
by it. They could argue, to the agency or in court, that
benign tumors should never be aggregated with malignant
tumors or that they should not be aggregated in a particular case. They might not convince the agency, but the
agency could not lawfully refuse to consider their arguments or reject evidence supporting them, and they might
convince a court that the agency guideline--i.e., its
choice of inference options--is wrong generally or inapplicable in a particular case.

If the guideline were an established agency procedure,
a private party could similarly argue that it is wrong
generally or inapplicable to a particular case. An
established procedure does not, therefore, preclude
efforts by third parties to treat the benign-versus-
malignant issue as an open question. The difference
between a recommendation and an established procedure
lies in the latter's effect on the agency itself. An
agency can depart from a recommendation at any time.
Under FDA's practice, however, it may not depart from an
established procedure unless it has previously announced
that it no longer regards the procedure as sound. In
other words, such an established procedure is binding on
the agency until formally revoked or changed, and third
parties can rely on it and insist that the agency adhere
to it.*

---

*The practical effects of the legal distinctions drawn
here are possibly overdrawn. The flexibility accorded by

There is another important difference between regulations and established procedures or, indeed, recommendations. To adopt regulations that have the reciprocally binding effects described above, an agency must follow the procedures prescribed by the Administrative Procedure Act, or by its own statute, for rule-making. At a minimum, these procedures include publication of a proposal, an opportunity for the submission of public comments, and promulgation of a final document that discusses and responds to all significant comments. The process can be long and acrimonious, and that helps to explain why agencies sometimes choose not to adopt policies, particularly those addressing complex issues, in the form of regulations. The same process must be followed to effect changes in regulations once adopted, and that inhibits rapid response to changes in scientific understanding.

ARGUMENTS FOR AND AGAINST THE USE OF GUIDELINES

The advantages and disadvantages listed below constitute an inventory of arguments that have been brought forward by the proponents and critics of guidelines for risk assessment. In most cases, an argument is most convincing for guidelines of a particular form and content, rather than for guidelines in general. For these cases, the characteristics of guidelines that would support or refute an argument are indicated.

---

any set of guidelines depends as much on the language chosen as on the legal form in which they appear. Suppose that an agency's default option is: "Ordinarily benign and malignant tumors shall be equated and their sum used to determine the significance of observed effects, unless (a) new data suggest the inappropriateness of this practice generally, or (b) results from the test in question or other tests of the compound make aggregation inappropriate in the particular case." This text anticipates exceptions, and would not prevent either the agency or a third party from taking a different view about the meaning of a particular test, whether it appeared as a regulation or in some other form.

ADVANTAGES OF GUIDELINE USE

Separation of Risk Assessment from Risk Management

Proponents of guidelines argue that their use would help
to separate risk assessment from other parts of the regulatory process. They contend that, when selected inference options are clearly delineated in a formal document,
risk assessments will not likely be influenced to fit
prior conclusions about regulation of a particular substance. The use of guidelines can also dispel the appearance of such influence when, in fact, there is none.
Agencies can defend their assessments on the grounds that
they always do them in the way set forth in the guidelines. Compared with reliance on the ad hoc selection of
inference options, the use of guidelines could reduce the
controversy focused on individual assessments. Debate
will shift to the more general discussion of the generic
choice of inference options addressed in the guidelines.
Guidelines that are comprehensive and detailed will define
and bracket the components of risk assessment most completely and explicitly. Thus, such guidelines could
probably provide the sharpest distinction between risk
assessment and risk management.

Quality Control

Proponents of guidelines argue that their use would ensure
the application of selected inference options based on the
informed judgment of experts. A single risk assessment
requires knowledge in diverse fields, such as epidemiology, biostatistics, toxicology, biochemistry, chemistry,
and clinical medicine. Generally, assessors have advanced
expertise in no more than a few fields. Guidelines could
help to bridge gaps in knowledge by ensuring that decisions are based on judgments formulated by experts in
each subject. Guidelines could also help to ensure that
assessors apply judgments that are in accord with current
scientific thinking in each field. This argument highlights the importance of including experts from a wide
range of scientific disciplines in the formulation of
guidelines. Furthermore, it suggests that guidelines
should be reviewed periodically so that new scientific
developments can be accommodated.
 Proponents believe that comprehensive, detailed guidelines would be most helpful in providing guidance to

assessors. Comprehensiveness is necessary to provide
guidance on all or most of the components of risk assessment. Detailed guidelines could provide an assessor with
an expert's insight into aspects of risk assessment that
require special consideration. How flexibility could
affect quality control is not clear; however, a flexible
framework could have a positive effect, especially if
guidelines can help an assessor to know when exceptional
or novel scientific evidence should be admitted.

Consistency

Almost all guideline documents have stated, in their
introductions, that consistency is a major rationale for
guideline use. Consistency in risk assessment is important to the agencies, because it helps to ensure fairness
and rationality by precluding the arbitrary application
of selected inference options that differ from one time
to the next. Consistency also permits comparison of risks
associated with different chemicals, and this is useful
for priority-setting and for facilitating regulatory
decision-making. When the same set of guidelines is
applied uniformly by all the agencies, government-wide
consistency may be improved. This has important implications for interagency coordination and for reducing the
possibility that risk assessments by different agencies
will be pitted against each other during litigation on a
given chemical. Guidelines of a type that fosters consistency among agencies have yet to be adopted and used. In
the absence of such guidelines, there are increased opportunities for inconsistency in the choice of inference
options available for each risk assessment component and
in the conclusions based on those choices. Proponents of
guidelines contend it is often difficult even to know
whether there is consistency among risk assessments,
because of lack of explicit documentation of inference
options used.
　　Comprehensive, detailed guidelines applied uniformly
across the agencies appear to be the most suitable form
for reducing inconsistency. To ensure thoroughness and
clarity in drawing conclusions, assessors should explicitly document the use of such guidelines in their reports.
Flexibility does not imply inconsistency in the application of risk assessment policy. The same inference
options can be applied consistently, except in instances
where convincing contrary scientific evidence is pre-

sented. When such evidence is available, the choice of different inference options has a scientific rationale and does not imply an arbitrary shift in risk assessment policy. It is not the same kind of inconsistency as that which can occur when, for example, one assessor uses a species-to-human conversion factor based on surface-area ratios and another, for no better scientific reason, uses a factor based on body-weight ratios.

Predictability

Proponents of guidelines argue that the private sector should be told explicitly which inference options the government will select to evaluate health-effects data. Industry needs this information to assess its own activities and testing programs. Without uniformly applied guidelines, a regulated party may have to call on the agencies for judgments on numerous issues and have no assurance that the judgments will not change unexpectedly or that one agency's judgment will be consistent with another's. Industry representatives have stated their preference for uniform federal guidelines (although they have been much more cautious in discussing the content of and legal weight given to the guidelines). Consider, for example, the following comment by the American Industrial Health Council, regarding the publication of the IRLG cancer guidelines (AIHC, 1979):

> The report is a significant step toward the formulation of a national cancer policy. AIHC supports the report's stated objective of ensuring that regulatory agencies evaluate carcinogenic risks consistently. We strongly urge that this initial step be followed up so that a national cancer policy is developed and conflicting policies among the regulatory agencies are minimized.

This point of view takes on added significance in view of the increasing desire of some states to develop their own cancer policies. Six states have initiated programs thus far, and California has already published its own guidelines (State of California, 1982a,b). For the private sector to have to contend with a range of different policies in different states would clearly be disadvantageous and burdensome. A federal cancer policy could serve as a model to the states and foster a more uniform approach to risk assessment.

Proponents believe that the most useful guidelines in gauging government actions would be detailed and comprehensive. Although flexibility may undermine predictability, it is reasonable to assume that industry would welcome such a trade-off. Guidelines published as established procedures would be the best option, for the regulatory agencies would not change their procedures without formal notice, but the procedures would not be binding on the regulated parties.

Evolutionary Improvement of the Risk Assessment Process

Proponents of guidelines argue that their use provides a locus for debate, examination, and revision of the selected inference options generally used in risk assessment. By contrast, the argument proceeds, when chemicals are evaluated on an ad hoc basis, the focus of debate is shifted from generic issues to case-specific issues, and the methods and assumptions of risk assessment are obscured from critical view.

Over the last decade, new and refined techniques of risk assessment have emerged. Two important examples are the use of short-term in vitro tests to infer carcinogenicity and mutagenicity and the use of dose-response assessment to estimate the magnitude of human risk at low doses. Guidelines may have contributed to the evolution of both by proposing generic interpretations that would be evaluated and tested both in theory and in the laboratory. The choice of a low-dose extrapolation model is a specific example. The first guidelines (FDA, 1973) proposed the use of the Mantel-Bryan model. This choice was the subject of much debate (FDA, 1977, 1979b); newer guidelines have suggested that this model has been discounted by the agencies, in part because it is essentially empirical and lacks biologic relevance with respect to current knowledge about carcinogenesis (IRLG, 1979b; EPA, 1980a). Furthermore, the debate over an appropriate model helped to foster a major research effort. The ED_{01} experiment, also known as the "megamouse study," involved the testing of 24,000 female mice given known carcinogens at low doses in an attempt to determine the shape of the response curve at low doses.

Guidelines that are comprehensive and detailed would invite the most opportunity for debate and evolutionary refinement.

Public Understanding

Because risk assessment is complex, it is easy to parody and demean the process. For example, the decision to label soft drinks containing saccharin was satirized in several highly publicized jokes, e.g., "Caution: Saccharin is hazardous to your rat" and "Drink 800 bottles of pop a day and get cancer." Proponents of guidelines argue that comprehensive, detailed guidelines setting forth the scientific and policy bases of risk assessment could improve public understanding and help to dispel the impression that government actions are based on tenuous and inadequate reasoning.

Administrative Efficiency

Some contend that when risk assessments are performed on a chemical-by-chemical basis without the use of guidelines, too many agency resources are devoted to reargument of the same issues with regulated parties. For example: Should animal carcinogenicity data be used to assess human risk? Should data on animals with a high incidence of spontaneous tumors be considered valid? Should benign tumors be assigned the same weight as malignant ones? Which statistical methods should be applied? Guidelines could reduce repetitious discussion by specifying which types of interpretations are acceptable, given the current state of scientific understanding.

OSHA, in its "Identification, Classification, and Regulation of Potential Carcinogens" (1980), registered concern about its efficiency (only seven rule-making proceedings completed in 9 years) and cited one major reason for its low productivity:

> The necessity to resolve basic scientific policy issues anew, in each rulemaking, has increased the burden on the Department of Labor and members of the scientific community called upon to address these widely accepted policies. Moreover, relitigation of these issues in the federal courts has also drained staff time and energy and has inhibited OSHA initiatives while its policy determinations were repeatedly relitigated.

OSHA maintained that the adoption of cancer guidelines was vital to efficient regulation:

> OSHA believes that this general policy and proce-
> dure will facilitate the sifting through the
> evidence concerning substances which may be
> interpreted to be potential carcinogens. . . .
> Without such a system and appropriate criteria,
> OSHA believes that this task cannot be accom-
> plished in a timely and efficient manner.

Efficiency could best be served by guidelines that are comprehensive, detailed, and inflexible and are adopted as regulations binding on all parties, but this would entail other costs. The disadvantages of such guidelines are described in some of the agruments cited in the following discussion.

DISADVANTAGES OF GUIDELINE USE

Oversimplification

The adoption of guidelines may foster a cookbook approach to risk assessment. The more assessors look at chemicals from a generic point of view, the less they are able to draw distinctions among them on the basis of specific data. The critics' ultimate concern is that blind adher- ence to guidelines might cause scientific information relevant to a particular chemical to be arbitrarily cast aside because it has not been accommodated in the guidelines.
The following underlined phrases are examples of guide- lines that critics believe may lead to oversimplification:

* <u>Use of the most sensitive species to determine risk</u>. Critics contend that, if information shows that metabolic similarity to humans is greater for a species that is less sensitive, data on this species may be preferable.
* <u>Absence of a threshold for carcinogenesis.</u> Critics argue that tumors may be induced by a genetic mechanism or by an epigenetic mechanism. In the latter case, a threshold may exist.
* <u>Unqualified acceptance of positive results at</u>

<u>high-dose testing</u>. Critics believe that validity should depend on whether there is a pharmacokinetic difference between high and low dose. Special consideration should be given to whether detoxifying or repair processes are saturated and to whether competing metabolic pathways are involved and become saturated.

Another potential problem is the lack of attention to weighting of evidence. For example, a guideline may simply state that "positive results in animal tests should always outweigh negative results." This does not take into account the quality and statistical power of the different tests; it could foster the attitude that such considerations are of minor importance.

To a large extent, the strength of such criticisms depends on the form and contents of the guidelines. Those which are comprehensive and leave little latitude for exceptional cases tend to maximize the problem of oversimplification; those which are flexible could be most effective in mitigating the problem. In addition, guidelines may explicitly direct the assessor to consider the weight of evidence of a given test result. For example, the IRLG guideline stated that positive results should supersede negative results, but added a caveat: "If the positive result is itself not fully conclusive or if reasons exist for questioning its validity as evidence of carcinogenicity, the result is generally classified as 'inconclusive' or 'only suggestive' even in the absence of other negative results."

Detailed guidelines can reduce the possibility of over-simplification if the intent of detail is to capture for the assessor the complexity of the issue addressed. For example, a guideline might state the scientific basis for the chosen inference option, the kinds of evidence that are typically applicable, circumstances in which accep-tance of exceptional evidence may be appropriate, and other rationales for choosing a particular inference option.

Regardless of the form of a guideline, there are some parts of risk assessment, particularly those dealing with the quality of data and the magnitude of uncertainty, that defy or at least resist generic interpretation. Individ-ual judgment is most important in such cases. A guide-line should not be viewed as a formula for producing risk assessments without the need for such judgment.

Mixing of Scientific Knowledge and Risk Assessment Policy

Guidelines unavoidably embody both scientific knowledge and risk assessment policy. In the past, regulatory agencies typically used a conservative approach in the development of risk assessment policy, as in the choice of the most sensitive species, use of the most conservative dose-response curve, and the lack of acceptance of negative epidemiologic data. Industry has been highly critical of this approach. Some representatives believe that risk assessment should be solely a scientific function and should be separated from policy decisions. Consider, for example, the American Industrial Health Council's criticism of the IRLG guidelines (AIHC, 1980):

> When the IRLG report speaks of the importance of using conservative methods or assumptions so as not to underestimate human risk, the report is mixing regulatory considerations into the scientific function. The scientific determination should be made separately from the regulatory determinations. On the basis of the best scientific estimate of the real risk, the regulatory agency can then consider costs, benefits and other elements that enter into a regulatory determination.

Furthermore, there is a fear that the mixing will go unrecognized outside the scientific community (AIHC, 1980):

> When value judgments are formalized by the selection, for "conservative" reasons, of a mathematical model or an assumption used for extrapolating human risk, the fact that value judgments have been made escapes the regulator and the public.

The first criticism appears to miss the crucial fact that risk assessment must always include policy, as well as science. The important issues are what the risk assessment policy content is and whether it will be applied consistently or not. The second criticism is most applicable to guidelines that permit an agency to represent as science the conclusions that have been reached in part on the basis of policy considerations. The argument is less applicable to guidelines that explicitly distinguish between scientific knowledge and risk assessment policy and direct the assessor to address such distinctions when reaching conclusions. Furthermore, it is not clear that risk assessment performed on an ad hoc basis would reduce the opportunity for unrecognized mixing of science and policy; indeed, carefully designed guidelines could help to inhibit such mixing.

Guidelines very different from the kinds described could be designed to be devoid of risk assessment policy choices. They would state the scientifically plausible inference options for each risk assessment component without attempting to select or even suggest a preferred inference option. However, a risk assessment based on such guidelines (containing all the plausible options for perhaps 40 components) could result in such a wide range of risk estimates that the analysis would not be useful to a regulator or to the public. Furthermore, regulators could reach conclusions based on the ad hoc exercise of risk assessment policy decisions.

Misallocation of Agency Resources to Development and Amendment of Guidelines

Critics contend that the dedication of time and resources to the process of guideline development and amendment detracts from an agency's ability to conduct regulatory activities. For example, OSHA's cancer guidelines required 3 years of effort before promulgation of the final rule in January 1980. The full rule-making record eventually exceeded 250,000 pages. OSHA itself offered some 45 witnesses who addressed the scientific content and the policy implications of the proposal, and a much larger number of witnesses appeared in behalf of other participants. The final policy consisted of more than 280 Federal Register pages of preamble and a dozen pages of regulatory text. Notwithstanding this intensive effort, the guidelines have yet to be applied, and new leadership at OSHA is in the process of reevaluating some provisions of the standard.

The procedures required by the Administrative Procedure Act are so elaborate that development and amendment of guidelines written as regulations are expected to demand more intensive effort than guidelines written as established procedures or recommendations. Regardless of the legal status given to the guidelines, their stability over time is susceptible to major changes in policy stances. However, guidelines that clearly distinguish scientific knowledge from risk assessment policy judgments could provide a locus for facilitating changes in policy orientation. They would define elements of risk assessment policy that are amenable to change and scientific elements that should not be changed for policy reasons. When risk assessment is done on an ad hoc basis, such distinctions may not exist.

Freezing of Science

Critics believe that guidelines would hinder the timely incorporation of important new scientific evidence during standard-setting. The Dow Chemical Company raised this concern about OSHA's cancer guidelines (OSHA, 1980):

> The record . . . has now made it clear that there is absolutely no assurance that the latest scientific evidence in the field will be permitted to be applied under the proposal to any given regulation of a specific chemical substance.

OSHA responded to this criticism by incorporating three amendment procedures into its cancer policy: a general review of the guidelines every 3 years by the directors of the National Cancer Institute, the National Institute of Environmental Health Sciences, and the National Institute for Occupational Safety and Health; recommendations at any time from the National Cancer Institute, the National Institute of Environmental Health Sciences, or the National Institute for Occupational Safety and Health; and petitions from the public. Final amendments would occur only through formal, independent rule-making, to ensure that major changes in the guidelines would not be made during the litigation of individual cases. In industry's perception, the amendment provision did not answer its initial criticism. The American Industrial Health Council characterized the amendment procedures as "a time-consuming and ponderous mechanism for incorporating into the regulatory standards newly available evidence or data concerning heretofore unresolved issues" (OSHA, 1980).

This argument is most applicable to guidelines that are adopted as regulations and to those which are comprehensive and inflexible. When guidelines are flexible and adopted as established procedures or recommendations, the rapid incorporation of novel scientific information is

more easily accommodated. The intent of flexibility is
to allow the acceptance of exceptional evidence based on
convincing scientific justification. In the case of
established procedures or recommendations, changes in
guidelines could occur without the necessity of a lengthy
rule-making process.

CONCLUSIONS

On the basis of its review of the historical record of
guideline development and use and its evaluation of the
arguments for and against guideline use, the Committee
has drawn several conclusions.

1. All agencies have found it necessary to write
guidelines, in part, to make their choice of inference
options more evident to the public. However, the application of inference options to specific risk assessments
has been marked by a general lack of explicitness.
Because of the lack of explicitness in identifying the
choice of inference options in specific risk assessments,
it has often been difficult to know whether assessors
adhere to guidelines. Within a given program, a consistent set of selected inference options may emerge over
time. However, the degree of consistency among programs
and agencies is not well defined.

2. Agency guidelines have varied markedly in form and
content. Without a deliberate coordinating effort, there
is no reason to assume that guidelines will become more
nearly uniform.
Although the scientific bases of cancer guidelines
developed in the past by the agencies have been generally
consistent, the degree to which the guidelines are comprehensive, detailed, flexible, and legally binding has
varied widely. EPA's guidelines are statements of broad
principles covering a few components in the four steps of
risk assessment; they have no regulatory status. OSHA's
guidelines were comprehensive and detailed and dealt
mainly with hazard identification; they were regulations.
CPSC's guidelines were not comprehensive and dealt mainly
with hazard identification; they had no regulatory status.
FDA's proposed sensitivity-of-method guidelines are comprehensive and detailed for dose-response assessment and
exposure assessment; they are regulations. The formation
of the IRLG caused the agencies to adopt a single set of

guidelines for the first time, but, since its disbanding
in 1981, there has been no further progress on guideline
development.*

3. <u>Uniform guidelines for risk assessment (except for
exposure assessment) are feasible and desirable.</u>
Guidelines are feasible. The Committee believes that
current statutory requirements would not prevent the use
of uniform guidelines. Regulators administer laws reflecting social policies that suggest different degrees of
acceptable risk. Some argue that uniform guidelines would
keep regulators from applying different standards of risk
that were based on these laws. However, regulators can
apply such standards on the basis of risk management
decisions after completion of the risk assessment. Furthermore, feasibility has already been demonstrated by
the adoption of the IRLG guidelines.

Uniform guidelines are desirable for several reasons.
First, the use of different guidelines by the agencies
could undermine the credibility of their risk assessments.
Critics of an agency risk assessment might argue persua-
sively that another agency estimates risk differently, on
the basis of a different set of inference options.
Second, almost every regulated chemical is in the jurisdiction of two or more agencies, and the possibility of
duplication of effort in performing risk assessments on a
given chemical could be minimized if the guidelines were
applied uniformly. Adoption of uniform guidelines could
foster joint risk assessment efforts by agencies interested in regulating the same chemical; or one agency could
rely on the assessment of another agency. Through such
cooperative efforts, a small agency like CPSC, which
lacks the scientific capability of EPA and FDA, could
gain help in evaluating complex data. Third, government-
wide guidelines could help industry to gauge government
actions and to define the types of data and interpretations relevant to industries' own testing programs.
Fourth, federal policy could orchestrate efforts toward
uniformity among the states.

---

*The Office of Science and Technology Policy (OSTP), with
agency participation, has written a document describing
the scientific basis of risk assessment. OSTP envisions
the ultimate evolution of a set of principles for risk
assessment from this document.

Exposure guidelines, in contrast with guidelines for other risk assessment steps, are not now readily amenable to uniform application in the various agencies. Apart from EPA, the agencies have rather narrowly defined interests regarding exposure, i.e., foods and drugs at FDA, consumer products at CPSC, and occupational hazards at OSHA. Whereas guidelines for the identification of hazard and for the quantitative estimation of risk in test animals may be commonly applied, no such common basis exists for applying exposure assessment guidelines.

4. Even well-designed guidelines may be unsuccessful unless:

- Attention is given to the process by which they are developed.
- They can accommodate change.
- They are viewed as valuable tools, rather than formulas for producing risk assessments.

Because guidelines must include both scientific knowledge and policy judgments, designing a development procedure is a difficult task. Risk assessment requires advanced knowledge in a number of disciplines, and guidelines should be formulated in part on the basis of the best possible scientific expertness in those disciplines. The best mechanism for determining risk assessment policy must be carefully defined. Because of the necessity of considering policy aspects in guidelines, duly appointed public officials must take responsibility for the policy implications. A major goal of the development process should be the assurance that the guidelines preserve a sharp distinction between scientific knowledge and risk assessment policy.

The Committee believes that guidelines should be capable of accommodating evolving scientific concepts in two ways. First, they should be periodically reviewed and, if necessary, revised. Second, they should permit acceptance of new evidence that differs from what was previously perceived as the general case, when scientifically justifiable. However, an unavoidable trade-off results from the use of such flexible guidelines: predictability and consistency may be reduced for the sake of flexibility.

Every risk assessment involves consideration of case-specific factors, such as the quality of the data or the overall strength of the evidence. These factors cannot

be addressed effectively in guidelines. If assessors
were to use guidelines in a strictly mechanical fashion,
without recognizing the importance of case-specific
judgments, the quality of risk assessments could be
diminished.

5. <u>Uniform guidelines for effects other than cancer
are desirable, but typically they would be based on a
less extensive scientific data base.</u>
The same reasons enunciated for the desirability of
cancer guidelines impel the conclusion that guidelines
are needed to guide assessments of other effects. Scientific data available on these effects may be organized to
provide useful information for assessing risk. In fact,
guidelines have already been developed for some of these
(although never adopted by the agencies), i.e., guidelines
for mutagenesis (EPA, 1980; March of Dimes Birth Defects
Foundation, 1981) and guidelines for reproductive and
teratogenic effects (ORNL/EPA, 1982; March of Dimes Birth
Defects Foundation, 1981).

REFERENCES

AIHC (American Industrial Health Council). October 17,
    1979. AIHC comments on: A Report of the Interagency
    Regulatory Liaison Group (IRLG), Work Group on Risk
    Assessment, entitled "Scientific Basis for Identifica-
    tion of Potential Carcinogens and Estimation of
    Risks," p. 2.
AIHC (American Industrial Health Council). April 30,
    1980. In Review of Public Comments on Statement on
    Regulation of Chemical Carcinogens; prepared for the
    U.S. Regulatory Council, Washington, D.C., pp. B-7,
    B-10.
CPSC (Consumer Product Safety Commission). 1978. Interim
    policy and procedure for classifying, evaluating, and
    regulating carcinogens in consumer products. Fed.
    Reg. 43:25658.
EPA (Environmental Protection Agency). April 5, 1972.
    Respondents brief in support of proposed findings,
    conclusions and order at 63-64, in re: Stevens Indus.,
    Inc. (consolidated DDT hearings).
EPA (Environmental Protection Agency). September 5,
    1975. Respondents motion to determine whether or not
    the registrations of mirex should be canceled or
    amended; Attachment A.

EPA (Environmental Protection Agency). 1976. Health
risk and economic impact assessments of suspected
carcinogens. Fed. Reg. 41:21402.

EPA (Environmental Protection Agency). 1980a. Mutagenicity risk assessments; proposed guidelines. Fed.
Reg. 45:74984.

EPA (Environmental Protection Agency). Office of Water
Regulations and Standards. 1980b. Water quality
criteria documents; availability. Fed. Reg.
45:79350-79353.

EPA (Environmental Protection Agency). Office of
Research and Development, Carcinogen Assessment
Group. August 8, 1980c. The Carcinogen Assessment
Group's method for determining the unit risk estimate
for air pollutants. External review copy, prepared
for Office of Air Quality Planning and Standards and
Office of Air, Noise and Radiation.

FDA (Food and Drug Administration). 1973. Chemical
compounds in food-producing animals; criteria and
procedures for evaluating assays for carcinogenic
residues. Fed. Reg. 38:19226.

FDA (Food and Drug Administration). 1977. Chemical
compounds in food-producing animals; criteria and
procedures for evaluating assays for carcinogenic
residues. Fed. Reg. 42:10412.

FDA (Food and Drug Administration). 1979a. Assessment
of Estimated Risk Resulting from Aflatoxins in
Consumer Product Peanut Products and Other Contaminants. Rockville, Md.: Food and Drug Administration.

FDA (Food and Drug Administration). 1979b. Chemical
compounds in food-producing animals; criteria and
procedures for evaluating assays for carcinogenic
residues. Fed. Reg. 44:17070.

FDA (Food and Drug Administration). 1982a. Code of
Federal Regulations, Title 21, Section 10.90.
Washington, D.C.: U.S. Government Printing Office.

FDA (Food and Drug Administration). 1982b. D & C Green,
No. 6, listing as a color additive in externally
applied drugs and cosmetics. Fed. Reg. 47:14138.

IRAC (International Agency for Research on Cancer). 1982.
General principles for evaluating the carcinogenic
risk of chemicals; in IARC monographs on the
Evaluation of the Carcinogenic Risk of Chemicals to
Humans. IARC, Lyon, France, vol. 29.

IRLG (Interagency Regulatory Liaison Group), Work Group
on Risk Assessment. 1979a. Scientific bases for
identification of potential carcinogens and estimation
of risks. Fed. Reg. 44:39858.

IRLG (Interagency Regulatory Liaison Group), Work Group
on Risk Assessment. 1979b. Scientific bases for
identification of potential carcinogens and estimation
of risks. J. Natl. Cancer Inst. 63:242.

Joint Food and Agricultural Organization and World Health
Organization Expert Committee on Pesticide Residues.
1965. Evaluation of the Toxicity of Pesticide
Residues in Food: Report of the 2nd Joint Meeting.
FAO Meet. Rep. No. PL/1965/10, WHO/Food Add./26.65.

Joint Food and Agricultural Organization and World Health
Organization Expert Committee on Food Additives.
1972. Evaluation of Certain Food Additives and the
Contaminants Mercury, Lead, and Cadmium. WHO Tech.
Rep. Ser. 505. Geneva.

Lehman, A. J., F. A. Vorhes, Jr., L. L. Ramsey, E. C.
Hagan, O. G. Fitzhugh, P. J. Schouboe, J. H. Draize,
E. I. Goldenthal, W. D'Aguanno, E. T. Lang, E. J.
Umberger, J. H. Gass, R. E. Zwickey, K. J. Davis, H.
A. Braun, A. A. Nelson, and B. J. Vos. 1959.
Appraisal of the Safety of Chemicals in Foods, Drugs
and Cosmetics. Association Food and Drug Officials of
the United States (AFDOUS).

March of Dimes Birth Defects Foundation. January 26-27,
1981. Guidelines for Studies of Human Populations
Exposed to Mutagenic and Reproductive Hazards;
Proceedings of Conference, Washington, D.C.

NRC/NAS (National Research Council/National Academy of
Sciences), Food Protection Committee, Food and
Nutrition Board. 1970. Evaluating the Safety of Food
Chemicals. Washington, D.C.: National Academy of
Sciences.

ORNL/EPA (Oak Ridge National Laboratory/Environmental
Protection Agency). February 1982. Assessment of
Risks to Human Reproduction and to Development of the
Human Conceptus from Exposure to Environmental
Substances. ORNL/EIS-197, EPA/9-82-001.

OSHA (Occupational Safety and Health Administration).
1977. Proposed rule: identification, classification
and regulation of potential occupational carcinogens.
Fed. Reg. 42:54148.

OSHA (Occupational Safety and Health Administration).
1980. Final rule: identification, classification and
regulation of potential occupational carcinogens.
Fed. Reg. 45:5001.

OSHA (Occupational Safety and Health Administration).
1981. Identification, classification and regulation
of potential occupational carcinogens; conforming
deletions. Fed. Reg. 46:4889.

OSHA (Occupational Safety and Health Administration).
1982. Identification, classification and regulation
of potential occupational carcinogens. Fed. Reg.
47:187.

OSTP (Office of Science and Technology Policy), Regulatory
Work Group on Science and Technology, Executive Office
of the President. October 1, 1982. Potential Human
Carcinogens: Methods for Identification and Characterization. Part 1: Current Views: Discussion Draft.

Regulatory Council. 1979. Statement on regulation of
chemical carcinogens: policy and request for public
comment. Fed. Reg. 44:60038.

State of California, Health and Welfare Agency. July
1982a. Carcinogen Identification Policy: A Statement
of Science as a Basis of Policy.

State of California, Health and Welfare Agency. October
1982b. Carcinogen Identification Policy: A Statement
of Science as a Basis of Policy; Section 2: Methods
for Estimating Cancer Risks from Exposures to
Carcinogens.

III
Organizational Arrangements for Risk Assessment

The different structures, procedures, and histories of the agencies responsible for regulating toxic substances have produced diversity in their approaches to risk assessment, but common patterns can be discerned, and they permit some broad generalizations about agency organizational arrangements.

First, most agencies have exerted little effort to maintain a sharp organizational separation between employees engaged in assessing the risks associated with substances and those responsible for identifying and evaluating regulatory responses. This is not to suggest that the same persons perform both functions; generally, they do not, for agency organizations reflect considerable specialization, recognizing the distinctive training and capabilities of staff members. However, the two functions are often housed in one organizational unit that is responsible for preparing integrated analyses that incorporate assessments both of risk and of recommended regulatory responses. Sometimes, risk assessment staff are employed in an office that is separate from the office of those who formulate and analyze regulatory options, but, with some notable exceptions, this organizational structure does not lead to a rigid separation of the two staffs.

Second, with the exception of a few experiments in interagency risk assessment during the late 1970s and continuing informal exchanges of information, each agency has performed its own assessments of the risks posed by substances that are candidates for regulation. This operational autonomy does not reflect willful ignorance of the activities of sister agencies or indifference to the desirability of consistency in the evaluation of common candidate substances. Rather, it is a product of several factors, including the lack of obvious mechanisms for formalized interagency collaboration, the desire of agency policy-makers to reserve authority for policy discretion in reaching conclusions based on risk assessment, the perception that the diversity of types of exposure for which each agency is responsible makes collaborative risk assessment impractical, and differences in regulatory priorities and schedules.

Third, although the four agencies have viewed themselves as ultimately responsible for the risk assessments that support their actions, they often extend their own staff resources available for performing risk assessment by relying on consultants and contractors who are closely supervised by agency personnel. Some agencies--notably the Occupational Safety and Health Administration (OSHA) and the National Institute for Occupational Safety and Health (NIOSH)--whose staffs are small or lack needed expertise rely very heavily on nongovernment contractors and outside scientists in the academic community and government research institutions for performance of risk assessments or specific tasks related to risk assessment (such as literature reviews).

In addition, outside scientists are often called on to review assessments produced by agency staff. Such consultations sometimes take place informally, but often through special advisory committees. These committees can be permanent, such as the Environmental Protection Agency (EPA) Clean Air Science Advisory Committee, or can be created to review particular risk assessments, as is done for many of the Food and Drug Administration (FDA) Bureau of Foods assessments. Some are established by statute, with requirements that they review agency assessments before regulations are proposed. Others are created voluntarily by an agency itself. The members of all federal advisory committees are appointed by the agencies, perhaps with the approval of higher executive-branch authority. Candidates for committee membership usually are identified by agency staff, although some agencies seek nominees from professional organizations and other interested parties. Nominations for some statutorily mandated committees are supplied by an external body, such as the National Academy of Sciences or the National Science Foundation. Advisory panels generally exercise considerable influence and, although legally they are only advisory, share to some extent the agencies' authority to reach conclusions about risk.

TABLE III-1 Examples of Four Models of Organizational Arrangements for Risk Assessment

Integration	Intra-agency Separation	Extra-agency Separation	Scientific Review Panels
OSHA Directorate of Health Standards Programs	EPA Carcinogen Assessment Group[a]	NIOSH-OSHA	EPA Scientific Advisory Panel
FDA Bureau of Foods		FDA Drug Evaluation Panels	EPA Science Advisory Board Subcommittee on Airborne Carcinogens
		Committees of the National Research Council	
		National Toxicology Program Panel on Formaldehyde[a]	

[a] Separate, centralized assessment body.

TYPES OF ORGANIZATIONAL ARRANGEMENTS

The prominent proposals for reforms in organizational structures and procedures for risk assessment have featured three interrelated principles:

* Risk assessment activities should be strictly separated from the analysis of risk management options and selection of regulatory strategies.
* Risk assessment activities should be centralized in a single body that serves all regulatory agencies.
* Expert panels composed of nonagency scientists should be used either to perform risk assessments for an agency or to review assessments developed by agency staff.

The Committee outlined four idealized models that reflect various combinations of these three principles. The models are integration, intra-agency separation (with or without centralization), extra-agency separation (with or without centralization), and use of scientific review panels. Examples of agency organizations that roughly approximate each model are identified below and in Table III-I. Most of the examples chosen have many distinctive characteristics that obscure or at least outweigh the three organizational principles. In addition, they are not the only examples of a particular model; others could have been reviewed.*

INTEGRATION

In this type of arrangement, a single organizational unit both performs risk assessments and develops regulations. In general, this arrangement is the most common for regulatory programs. For example, for the assessment of chronic hazards involved with chemicals from consumer products, the Consumer Product Safety Commission (CPSC)

---

*The Committee considered the possible merits of reviewing risk assessment procedures used by other countries as well and decided not to pursue this line of investigation, because of the great differences in political and institutional structures between this country and other countries. Such differences would make it very difficult, if not impossible, to extrapolate findings on institutional structures used in other countries to the United States.

Directorate for Health Sciences is the responsible unit.
Before 1977, the Directorate for Health Sciences had few
people involved in the risk assessment process, and risk
assessments as such were not generally used. Since then,
the Directorate has acquired the expertise needed to perform risk assessments itself. The risk assessment is
performed within the Directorate, which is distinct from
the Commission's politically appointed policy decision-
makers. Two different examples of this model examined by
the Committee are the OSHA Directorate of Health Standards
Programs and the FDA Bureau of Foods (Table III-1). In
the former example, risk assessors and those responsible
for formulating and recommmending regulatory strategies
are in the same organizational unit. FDA's Bureau of
Foods has a separate office that performs risk assessment,
but this separation stems from a functional division of
scientific disciplines; it is not intended to and does
not result in formal separation of the risk assessment
staff from the regulatory staff.

INTRA-AGENCY SEPARATION

In this model, risk assessment is performed by a group
that is ostensibly separate from and independent of the
office responsible for regulation in the same agency. An
intra-agency risk assessment unit could be program-
specific or agency-wide. There are examples of program-
specific, organizationally separate risk assessment units
(notably the Environmental Criteria and Assessment Offices
in EPA), but the Committee did not examine them; instead,
it reviewed activities of the EPA Carcinogen Assessment
Group as an example of an internally separate, agency-
wide body.

EXTRA-AGENCY SEPARATION

In this model, an agency's risk assessment is developed
outside the agency. The examples reviewed demonstrate
the wide variety of arrangements included in this model.
Full organizational separation can be achieved by having
one institution perform risk assessment and a separate
institution regulate exposure to hazardous substances.
The relation between NIOSH and OSHA was studied as an
example of a permanent, statutory arrangement of this
kind. A regulatory agency's use of expert panels to

perform risk assessments can also result in extra-agency
separation of risk assessment and regulation. Committees
of the National Research Council and several groups of
panels used by FDA to review the safety and effectiveness
of drugs provide varied examples of such arrangements.
The National Toxicology Program Panel on Formaldehyde is
an example of an ad hoc assessment group that consisted
of government scientists, was organizationally separate
from the regulatory agencies (although not without agency
members), and served all four agencies (i.e., it was
centralized). Because the Interagency Regulatory Liaison
Group did not perform risk assessments, it has not been
examined as an example of an extra-agency assessment body.

USE OF SCIENTIFIC REVIEW PANELS

Agencies may use independent scientific panels to perform
risk assessments or to review assessments prepared by the
agencies. This distinction has been used by the Committee
to facilitate separate discussion of panels that perform
assessments as examples of full organizational separation
(see preceding discussion) and panels that review agency
assessments as examples of independent review panels.
However, the dichotomy is somewhat artificial, in that
there may be difficulty in classifying a particular panel.
For example, if a panel responsible for performing risk
assessments comes to rely heavily on preliminary analyses
prepared by agency staff, it can be thought of as acting
in a review capacity. Conversely, panels assembled solely
for the purpose of reviewing agency assessments have often
displayed remarkable independence, sometimes preparing
long critiques of agency documents and suggesting substitute findings and reasons. In such cases, to specify
which group had performed and which had reviewed the
agency's final assessment of risk is difficult.

The extent to which agencies have used independent
scientific panels has varied considerably. For example,
OSHA has available two types of advisory committees:
standing bodies, such as the National Advisory Committee
on Occupational Safety and Health, and ad hoc committees
that provide advice on specific standards. Members of
both types of committee are expected to be knowledgeable
about occupational safety and health and may include
persons mainly interested in law or regulatory policies.
In addition to their professional expertise, however,
members of OSHA committees are intended to be represen-

tative of groups interested in occupational health and safety. Several committees have reviewed risk assessments prepared by OSHA or NIOSH. However, because members were intended to be representatives of interest groups, reviews were usually forums for policy debates, not scientific evaluations of risk assessments. In its initial years, OSHA routinely appointed an advisory committee for each regulatory proceeding.

CPSC has had the least experience with expert panels. Before 1981, the Commission was not required to have any assessment of carcinogenic hazard reviewed by an outside panel, although it did make occasional use of such panels (most notably CPSC's request for the National Toxicology Program to form a panel on formaldehyde). CPSC's reauthorization in 1981 included a provision that, before any regulatory action could be proposed on a substance potentially presenting a carcinogenic, teratogenic, or mutagenic hazard, a chronic hazard advisory panel (CHAP) must be established, with the cooperation of the National Academy of Sciences, to review the toxicity of the substance. The first CHAP has recently been convened to review the toxicity of asbestos. Thus, CPSC relies on two methods of peer review for any proposed action. First, independent peer review by outside experts, as well as by a scientific review panel, is performed before a notice of proposed rule-making is issued. Second, the Commission relies on a public rule-making proceeding in accordance with the Administrative Procedure Act during which comment is invited through a Federal Register notice on all aspects of the proposed action. Extensive written comments have been received in the past by this procedure, from industry, consumer groups, members of the academic and scientific communities, and others. Additionally, open, informal public hearings may be held in which interested groups present their views orally; in the past, several such hearings were held during the consideration of a single substance (formaldehyde).

FDA has often used independent scientific panels both to perform and to review agency assessments. The Bureau of Drugs has used standing committees to review and evaluate data on the safety and effectiveness of drug products and to make appropriate recommendations to the Commissioner (see preceding discussion). The use of independent panels by the Bureau of Foods, however, has been on an ad hoc basis, usually at the agency's discretion. However, there are exceptions; for example, the Food, Drug, and Cosmetic Act requires that carcinogenicity issues related to color additives be referred to a committee of experts selected by the National Academy of Sciences.

EPA, in contrast, has had less choice in its relations with its advisory committees. Several statutes require EPA to consult such committees for scientific review of agency risk assessments or regulations. Examples of mandated advisory committees with a primarily scientific role include the Agency-wide Science Advisory Board; the Clean Air Scientific Advisory Committee, a part of this Board, which reviews criteria documents for air-quality standards; and the Scientific Advisory Panel, which focuses on scientific issues in the Agency's Office of Pesticide Programs. The Committee has examined this panel and a subcommittee of the Science Advisory Board as examples of scientific review panels.

Agency actions, including risk assessments, have been reviewed in the Executive Office of the President; however, because these reviews have, with a few notable exceptions, focused primarily on risk management concerns, the Committee has not examined them.

REVIEW OF AGENCY PROCEDURES FOR RISK ASSESSMENT

This section describes the practices used for risk assessment in each of the organizational examples reviewed by the Committee. The descriptions that follow reveal some strengths and weaknesses of particular approaches and permit some tentative generalizations to be made. Such generalizations, augmented by the experience and judgment of Committee members, lead in turn to recommendations applicable to organizational arrangements for the performance of risk assessment.

The Committee's necessarily retrospective review of agency performance has focused on events and practices of the 1970s, which triggered the current proposals for reform. Changes have been implemented, or at least are contemplated, in the procedures of several of the agencies studied, and the Committee recognized that such changes could alter the performance of risk assessment. Some of the descriptions of agency practices presented here may be dated. However, our purpose is not to describe the current organizational structure of agencies, but rather to discern in the historical record any general relationships between organizational design and procedures and the quality of risk assessments. The paucity of experience with recent organizational changes and the tendency of any new administration to disclaim the approaches of predecessors while proclaiming the effectiveness of reforms make very recent history less germane to the Committee's purpose.

OSHA'S DIRECTORATE OF HEALTH STANDARDS PROGRAMS (DHSP)

OSHA's health standards were expected by Congress to be based on criteria and recommended standards provided by NIOSH. However, improvements in OSHA's scientific capability and a court directive that OSHA itself review all studies included in the risk assessment supporting a proposed standard prompted the agency to rely less heavily on NIOSH and to begin performing its own risk assessments. Until 1976, OSHA had only a few personnel in the health sciences; however, DHSP has since become an organization staffed primarily by health professionals, including industrial hygienists, responsible for performing risk assessments and for preparing standards, relying on economic and technical analyses supplied by the Office of Regulatory Analysis in a separate directorate (Figure III-1). In addition, the Directorate normally has used a number of consultants who assist with risk assessment or other aspects of standard development, contributing considerable specialized expertise to the organization.

OSHA tried to achieve organizational separation of risk assessment from the preparation of standards in the case of carcinogens. One office in DHSP was supposed to do risk assessment, another to draft standards. In practice, however, such separation was not achieved, largely because personnel shortages required that individual staff members perform both functions.

Agenda and Procedures

DHSP's regulatory and risk assessment agenda has been determined largely by two external forces: petitions by labor unions for action on particular hazards and dramatic discoveries of previously unidentified workplace hazards. Court remands of several OSHA standards, such as the benzene standard, provided new work for OSHA, but none of the mandated re-examinations has led to a final standard. Criteria documents prepared by NIOSH also contributed to OSHA's agenda, in that DHSP staff always read these docu-

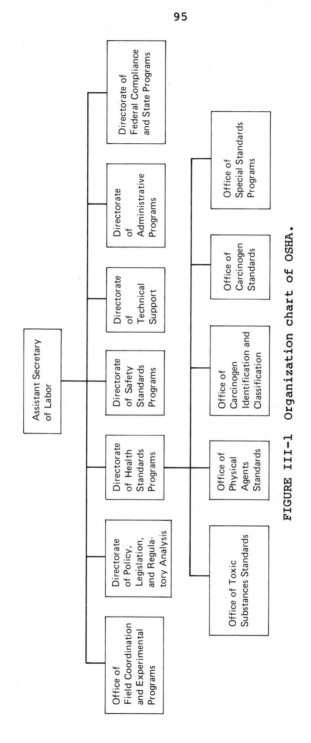

FIGURE III-1 Organization chart of OSHA.

ments when they were received and normally published a
Federal Register notice soliciting further information.
DHSP's risk assessments usually began with a NIOSH
criteria document or other NIOSH input, whatever information was submitted with a labor petition if there was
one, the data available from any precipitating discovery,
and assessments performed by others, such as the National
Academy of Sciences. A literature search and review were
conducted by DHSP personnel, often with the help of consultants and NIOSH personnel; and sometimes environmental
data on the workplace were solicited or obtained by
contractors to contribute to the exposure assessment.

DHSP has not prepared special assessment documents
before issuing notices of proposed rule-making. Thus,
the first indication provided to the public of the results
of an OSHA risk assessment and of the conclusions it
intended to draw therefrom was in the Federal Register
preamble to its proposed standard. Public comment was
invited on all aspects of the proposed standard, including the risk assessment. Extensive written comments were
usually received from industry, labor, and others, such
as members of the academic scientific community. Customarily a hearing was held at which oral presentations
were made and at which questioning of witnesses by OSHA
personnel and other witnesses was permitted. The preamble
to the final rule, if one were issued, included OSHA's
final risk assessment, which incorporated a literature
review and OSHA's conclusions on the available scientific
data.

In 10 years, OSHA produced permanent health standards
for 23 substances or processes, 14 of which were regulated together in a single rule-making. OSHA has also
proposed standards for eight substances for which final
standards have never been issued, and assessments were
conducted for several substances for which new or updated
standards are now being considered (Table III-2).

Methods and Use of Guidelines

For most of its history, OSHA has not had formal guidelines for carcinogenic risk assessment. Instead, agency
staff have conducted their assessments by choosing options
for the components of risk assessment on a case-by-case
basis. However, the generic guidelines for identification and classification of carcinogens proposed in 1977
and revised and promulgated in 1980 were intended to

TABLE III-2   A Summary of OSHA Standards

Standards Completed	Standards Proposed, But Not Completed	Standards Being Developed
Asbestos	Arsenic[a]	Ethylene oxide
Vinyl chloride	Beryllium	Asbestos
Arsenic[a]	Sulfur dioxide	Ethylene dibromide
Benzene	Ketones	Cotton dust, nontextile sectors
Coke-oven emission	Hearing conservation (noise)	
14 carcinogens	Toluene	
Lead	Ammonia	
Cotton dust	MOCA	
1,2-Dibromo-3-chloropropane	Trichloroethylene	
Acrylonitrile		

[a]The arsenic standard was remanded to OSHA by the Court of Appeals for the Ninth Circuit for purposes of making a significant-risk determination consistent with the Supreme Court's benzene decision.

replace criteria used in individual cases with generic guidelines that would be applied consistently to all risk assessments of potential carcinogens. The choices incorporated in the 1980 cancer policy reflected the policy orientations of incumbent senior agency officials. Changes now contemplated in these guidelines reflect the policy orientation of the current OSHA management. Similarly, although for many years OSHA did not perform quantitative risk estimates for use in setting standards for carcinogens, it now intends to do so where appropriate. This change results from policy decisions of senior agency officials, based, at least in part, on their interpretation of the Supreme Court's decision on benzene. (Agency officials have interpreted the decision to mean that quantitative dose-response assessments should be

performed for individual substances if data are
sufficient.)

Peer Review

OSHA historically has done a less thorough job than other
agencies in obtaining relevant scientific information
and independent peer review of this information before
issuing a notice of proposed rule-making. Instead, the
agency has relied primarily on the public rule-making
proceeding to identify new information, much of which is
in the possession of interested parties and is unlikely
to be brought forward except in the context of rule-
making. Similarly, although NIOSH's and OSHA's initial
assessments often did not provide a critical review of
relevant data, critiques of this information were given
to the agency during rule-making proceedings, and the
agency's final assessment of the risks posed by a chemical often was substantially changed as a result. OSHA's
use of rule-making proceedings to provide scientific
review stands in sharp contrast with the other agencies'
procedures for review. In the Committee's opinion, this
reliance on public proceedings to strengthen and refine
the scientific basis for the agency's regulatory actions
has not been an adequate substitute for independent peer
review. In addition, reliance on public proceedings
surely precipitated some of the criticism of agency
actions and may have jeopardized the scientific integrity
and procedural legitimacy of the agency's risk assessments.
     Although OSHA's standard-setting actions have stimu-
lated intense controversy, much of it has focused on
issues separate from risk assessment. Questions of costs
and technologic feasibility (risk management issues) have
stimulated much debate. Discussions of the agency's risk
assessments have usually focused on its conclusions and
their relationship to the agency's regulatory mandate,
rather than on its characterization of risk. When OSHA's
risk assessments were challenged during rule-making, some
key subjects of contention were OSHA's adherence to the
assumption that carcinogens have no threshold for causing
adverse effects, its tendency to give positive data
greater weight than negative data, its use of single epidemiologic studies to support regulatory action, the
validity of specific experiments and the agency's interpretation of the data from them, and the decision as to

whether quantitative assessments of risk should be considered. These issues, of course, have both policy and scientific implications.

FDA'S BUREAU OF FOODS

The Food and Drug Administration enforces the Federal Food, Drug, and Cosmetic Act and several related statutes. Its jurisdiction ranges from basic foods to the most advanced pharmaceuticals and medical equipment. The agency assesses the risks associated with thousands of new and existing products every year, functioning through product-oriented units whose responsibilities are reflected in their titles: Foods, Drugs and Biologics, Veterinary Medicine, and Devices and Radiological Health (Figure III-2). The bureaus' agendas are dictated both through internal planning and by external events, particularly applications for approval of new products. Because the Bureau of Foods has had considerable experience with products that pose potential cancer risks, the Committee has focused on this part of FDA in its review.

Agenda and Procedures

The Bureau's risk assessment functions fall into three broad categories: review of petitions for marketing of new compounds for which the manufacturer provides supporting toxicologic and exposure (or use) data; planned retrospective or cyclic review of approved compounds, supporting data on which the Bureau generally must take as it finds them; and review of inadvertent contaminants in food, supporting data on which are derived from many sources, including open scientific literature, monographs, reports, manufacturers' data, and agency-generated data.

In 1981, the Bureau of Foods evaluated 65 food additives, two color additives, and approximately 45 animal-drug petitions. These totals, however, do not reveal the total number of Bureau inquiries that could qualify as risk assessments, albeit perfunctory. Each time a new contaminant is discovered, for example, the Bureau performs some assessment of the risks, although the available data are often limited and little time is available to gather data before it must decide whether to initiate control measures. Similarly, every reported change in

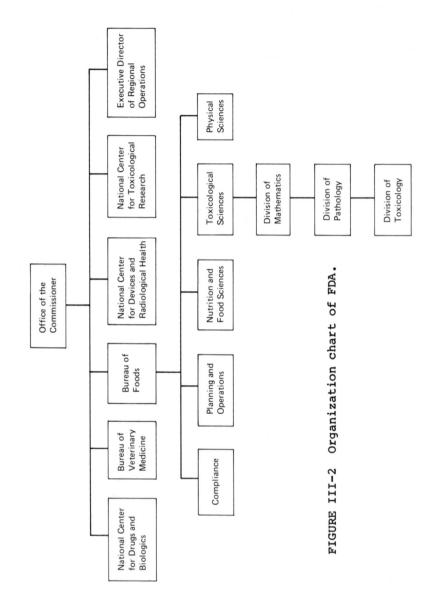

FIGURE III-2 Organization chart of FDA.

degree of contamination invites a new risk assessment.
As one would predict, the time and effort required vary
with the context. The Bureau's procedures for reviewing
food additives, color additives, and residues of animal
drugs are more routine than those for evaluating food
contaminants, whose occurrence is largely unpredictable.
On receipt in the Division of Food and Color Additives, a
food-additive petition is evaluated to determine whether
it is acceptable for filing. This involves not only
review of its formal adequacy, but a preliminary assessment of the toxicologic data to determine whether all
potential health effects have been studied.

After official filing of the petition, scientists from
the appropriate divisions (ordinarily with the assistance
of scientists outside the agency) study the supporting
chemical, toxicologic, and exposure data to decide whether
the compound is safe. The food-additive law has been
construed as requiring, even when the Delaney clause is
not applicable, "reasonable certainty" that no consumer
will be harmed. No effort is made to evaluate the benefits that an additive might provide, but the Bureau must
be satisfied that the additive achieves its intended
effects. This exercise usually has two parts: first,
Division of Toxicology scientists determine a no-observed-
effect concentration for the additive on the basis of
acute, subchronic, and chronic feeding studies in animals;
second, applying a so-called safety factor, they determine
a permissible extent of use in human food or an acceptable
daily intake. This value is then compared with the estimated daily human exposure based on the manufacturer's
proposed use and predicted human consumption of the foods
in which the additive is to be used. An acceptable exposure to an additive is one at which human exposure is at
or below the acceptable daily intake. Under current law,
this intake value cannot be established for a direct food
or color additive that is carcinogenic; such a substance
may not be approved for use.

The risk assessment function is performed entirely by
Bureau scientists. Bureau staff, including the reviewing
scientists, may meet with representatives of the peti-
tioner to discuss uncertainties, request additional data,
or suggest reduced use. Typically, both the scientific
and the regulatory aspects of food-additive petitions are
reviewed and resolved at the division level in the Bureau
of Foods. On petitions that raise difficult scientific
and policy issues or that pose the question of carcinogenicity, the divisions generally seek advice or direction

from the associate directors, Bureau deputy directors, or
the Bureau Director. The Bureau may, in turn, seek advice
from the Chief Counsel, from other bureaus, or from the
Commissioner's office during the review of petitions that
present particular scientific, legal, or policy questions.

Once the responsible unit is satisfied that an additive
is approvable and thus that a regulation is appropriate,
the Division of Food and Color Additives prepares a document package consisting of an action memorandum, a draft
Federal Register document, and supporting material, which
is then forwarded through established review channels to
the Director's office for final Bureau approval and trans-
mission to the Commissioner's office. The action memorandum recommending approval by the Associate Commissioner
for Regulatory Affairs, to whom the Commissioner has dele-
gated formal approval authority, necessarily incorporates
both scientific assessments and regulatory judgments.
Because the governing legal standard focuses exclusively
on the health effects of the additive, the approval process is not influenced by consideration of economic or
other benefits.

The sequence of analysis in the Bureau for environmental contaminants does not differ sharply from that
described above for food additives, although different
divisions may participate in the process and economic
factors are consciously considered. The statutory provision under which FDA regulates food contaminants contemplates that it will balance the risk posed by a substance
against the effects of reducing consumer exposure, such
as loss of food and increases in price. Accordingly, the
action memorandum sent to the Bureau Director recommends
an exposure limit based on three criteria: an assessment
of the risk posed by the contaminant, an evaluation of
available methods of chemical analysis to monitor its
presence, and an estimate of the economic effects of
alternative limits.

Methods and Use of Guidelines

Although the Bureau's approach to the evaluation of acute
toxicants has remained stable over a long period, its
methods for evaluating potential carcinogens have under-
gone substantial change since the early 1970s. In 1978,
the Bureau Director formed a Cancer Assessment Committee
in the Office of Toxicological Sciences to evaluate the
carcinogenicity of substances being considered for

approval or regulation and to perform risk assessments.
A list of substances reviewed by this Committee in 1981
is given in Table III-3. The 12 members of the Committee
are all FDA employees and include toxicologists, pathol-
ogists, mathematicians, and chemists. The role of the
Committee is to render all final decisions on carcinogenicity for the Bureau of Foods on the basis of scientific information available to it. Its primary function
is to determine whether, on the basis of a fair evaluation of all available data, a chemical is a potential or
actual carcinogen. Because the Delaney clause, which
forbids exposure of any food or color additive that
induces cancer, applies to many substances in the Bureau's
jurisdiction, quantitative (e.g., dose-response) assessments are not always performed. For some substances, such
as contaminants, the magnitude of the risk is relevant,
and scientists from the various divisions collaborate with
staff responsible for gathering information on human exposure to perform risk characterizations. The Cancer
Assessment Committee does not typically prepare formal
written assessments, so there is no document available
that outlines the relevant data and the rationale for the
choices of options made in the assessment of risks. The
Cancer Assessment Committee apparently does not follow
comprehensive written guidelines, although it does follow
some general guidelines that were used in previous decisions and are set out in the agency's drug-residue
proposal.

Peer Review

In recent years, the Bureau of Foods has sought independent scientific review of the data on a number of substances. Often Bureau staff informally solicit the judgments of individual outside scientists on major issues.
The Bureau routinely uses outside panels established
under the auspices of the Federation of American Societies
for Experimental Biology for periodic review of substances
now generally recognized as safe (GRAS). Ad hoc panels
were convened to evaluate the data on such substances as
cyclamate, saccharin, Red No. 2, and Red No. 40.
     More recently, the Bureau has turned to a standing
panel, the Board of Scientific Counselors of the National
Toxicology Program. The Board's review of the data on
color additive Green No. 5 illustrates the Bureau's
approach to external peer review. The Board reviewed the

TABLE III-3   Substances Evaluated for Carcinogenicity by
the FDA Cancer Assessment Committee in 1981

Acrylonitrile	1,2-Dichloroethane
Lead acetate	Diethylhexylphthalate
Vinyl chloride	Diethylhexyladipate
Dioxane	Furazolidone
p-Toluidine	Cinnamyl anthranilate
Hydrazine	Trimethylphosphate

original data from a study done by a commercial laboratory, which were submitted with a petition for approval
of the substance. The Board also considered aspects of
the analysis done by Bureau staff and conducted an independent evaluation of the pathology slides and a statistical analysis of the study results. Bureau scientists
asked that the Board reach a conclusion concerning the
strength of the evidence of carcinogenicity. Thus, the
Board was limited to scientific issues and did not consider the possible social implications of its finding.
After the Board's finding that the evidence was inconclusive and before the Bureau's conclusion that the
additive was unlikely to be a human carcinogen, Bureau
staff performed a risk characterization to estimate the
potential risks if this conclusion were in error.
   The decision to consult an outside panel for review of
risk assessments for potential carcinogens is made by the
Chairman of the Cancer Assessment Committee. The Bureau
currently is considering establishing a standing committee that could be called on to review agency assessments.
It is likely that the impetus to form a standing review
committee stems from criticisms of past agency practices,
especially those followed in the evaluation of the data
on nitrite. In this instance, FDA's contemplated action
against nitrite in 1979 was announced before Bureau scientists had had an opportunity to evaluate the critical
toxicity data and to refer the data to an independent
panel. This controversial chapter in FDA's history of
regulating food ingredients has often been cited as
demonstrating the need for systematic peer review of the
agency's risk analyses in order to avoid the problems
that can arise when risk management considerations affect
the conduct of risk assessments. The existence of a
standing panel, although no guarantee, may discourage

agency officials from deviating from standard Bureau procedures that are now designed to ensure adequate peer review.

EPA'S CARCINOGEN ASSESSMENT GROUP

EPA's Carcinogen Assessment Group (CAG) was created in 1976 by the EPA Administrator to implement generic and uniform agency guidelines for carcinogenic risk assessment. Initially, it was a separate body in the Agency's Office of Research and Development and reported directly to its Assistant Administrator. In 1979, however, the Office of Health and Environmental Assessment was established in the Office of Research and Development, and CAG became one of several assessment groups (Figure III-3). Organizationally, CAG staff are separate from, and independent of, the risk management function; i.e., it is an example of intra-agency separation. It also serves as an example of an internally centralized assessment body, in that it performs assessments for several different regulatory programs in EPA.

Although CAG personnel do meet and talk with regulatory program personnel and are customarily well aware of any programmatic interest in particular substances and of interest-group preferences, this office is insulated from the day-to-day pressures of program offices. Thus, the organizational arrangement that places CAG in the Office of Research and Development does have the initial effect of freeing risk assessment personnel from specific policy issues that arise when risk management options are considered. However, when a scientific review committee examines documents produced by this office later in the process, interest groups are able to express their views and CAG personnel are no longer isolated from such influences.

Currently, all CAG assessments are done by in-house staff, although in the past some were done by consultants. Usually, contractors are employed only for the time-consuming and mechanical task of conducting literature searches. Responsibility for each assessment is assigned to a particular person, but other staff members contribute to various sections according to their particular specialties and expertness. Its staff has been remarkably stable; since 1976, only one person has left the group. As of October 1982, 11 full-time professionals were on its staff, nine of whom had doctorates. Most staff members have an academic background, and their professional work experience averages 10 years. The staff includes

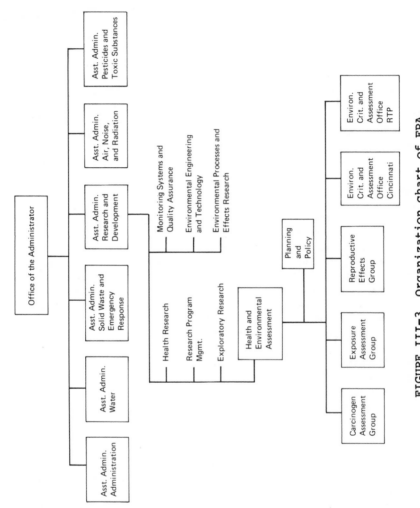

FIGURE III-3 Organization chart of EPA.

three biostatisticians, two biochemists, two epidemiologists, one biophysicist, one pathologist, one pharmacologist, and one endocrinologist. The former Director, now a consultant, is the only physician associated with the office.

Agenda and Procedures

CAG does not initiate its own assessments; instead, it responds to requests from regulatory (program) offices in EPA. It does, however, set its own priorities in consultation with the program offices, on the basis of the workload of requests and the urgency of the need for the assessments. Although it serves as a risk assessment body for the whole Agency, not all programs in EPA use CAG. The most notable exception is the Office of Toxic Substances. Apparently, one factor cited by program offices as leading to this lack of use is the length of time CAG requires to complete an assessment.

Since 1976, CAG has prepared assessments for approximately 150 chemicals. The length and scope of the documents produced vary with the data available, with their purpose, and with the needs of the requesting office. They can range from brief and preliminary literature reviews relevant to hazard identification or tentative estimates of risk as a function of dose to complete and thorough literature reviews leading to a comprehensive risk characterization. In-depth evaluations may or may not include quantitative dose-response assessments. As an example of its work agenda, CAG has covered 41 chemicals for the Agency's Office of Air Quality Planning and Standards. In-depth evaluations were performed for nine (see Table III-4), and preliminary assessments for 32.

Methods and Use of Guidelines

The risk assessments performed by this group are based on Agency guidelines developed initially by CAG in 1976 for use by the entire Agency. These guidelines have been revised after initial publication, and some of the changes have also been published (EPA, 1979, 1980). Normally, individual assessment documents produced do not reexamine or indeed articulate underlying guidelines; rather, the reader is presumed to know that EPA and CAG rely on guidelines that embody particular choices among several

TABLE III-4 Substances Fully Evaluated by the Carcinogen
Assessment Group for the EPA Office of Air Quality
Planning and Standards

Arsenic	Methyl chloroform[a]
Benzene	Methylene chloride[a]
Vinyl chloride	Tetrachloroethylene[a]
Acrylonitrile[a]	Trichloroethylene[a]
Coke-oven emission[a]	

---

[a]Under review as of October 1982.

inference options available. Also, the changes made in
the guidelines have not, in many cases, been formally
acknowledged; i.e., the current guidelines do not exist
in a single publicly accessible written document. CAG's
use of guidelines, especially for hazard identification,
has been regarded by some EPA review panels--notably, the
Subcommittee on Airborne Carcinogens--as too inflexible,
possibly misleading, and interfering with critical analysis of underlying data. In fact, the initial published
guidelines (EPA, 1976) did permit different interpretations of data and the use of different risk assessment
methods; however, the methods embodied in CAG assessments
and those related to dose-response assessment and published in EPA's Water Quality Methodology for Carcinogens
do not reflect this flexibility. The misunderstandings
experienced with the Subcommittee on Airborne Carcinogens
(and other review bodies) have stemmed to a great degree
from the facts that CAG's guidelines are in flux, remain
unwritten, and are not presented in the individual
assessment documents provided to the review committees.
As a result, reviewers are likely to be unaware of the
operational ground rules used in interpreting carcinogenicity data and developing risk estimates. The absence
of an explicit discussion of the application of Agency
guidelines and of discussion of the rationale for the
choices made in a risk assessment blurs the distinction
between science and policy considerations in CAG
assessments.

Peer Review

Drafts are reviewed by all members of the CAG staff and its Director. Drafts are also usually sent for review on an ad hoc basis to knowledgeable persons outside the agency. However, this review process is not part of the public record, and criticism may be accepted or rejected at CAG's discretion. The lack of adequate procedures to ensure that peer review comments are given proper consideration may lessen any benefits to be derived from peer review early in the process of developing a risk assessment. Draft risk assessments are usually reviewed by the Director of the Office of Health and Environmental Assessment, directors of other units in this office, and Office of Research and Development staff before being submitted to the requesting program office. CAG assessments are often submitted to committees of EPA's Science Advisory Board or to the Scientific Advisory Panel for peer review. Such reviews take place in public sessions, in accordance with the requirements of the Federal Advisory Committee Act. They provide an opportunity for interested members of the public to review CAG documents and to communicate criticisms to the reviewing committee and EPA. Reviews of CAG assessments by EPA panels have been mixed, with some panels, such as the Scientific Advisory Panel, often approving the assessments and others finding numerous shortcomings related to both substance and format (e.g., the Subcommittees on Arsenic as a Possible Hazardous Air Pollutant and on Airborne Carcinogens of the Agency's Science Advisory Board). This public review process usually leads to revisions.

NIOSH-OSHA

The Occupational Safety and Health Act of 1970 created two new organizations: OSHA and NIOSH. OSHA was a new component of the Department of Labor. NIOSH was placed in the Department of Health, Education, and Welfare, now the Department of Health and Human Services. Since 1973, NIOSH has been a part of the Centers for Disease Control in the U.S. Public Health Service. The common mission set for both agencies was the protection of the health of American workers. NIOSH's primary functions included the conduct of research and development of criteria for recommendations to OSHA for occupational health standards. In addition, the Act authorized NIOSH to "develop and establish recommended occupational safety and health standards." Although it is not technically correct to refer to NIOSH criteria documents simply as risk assessments, because the documents contain additional information concerning risk management (e.g., engineering considerations) as well as recommended standards, the documents normally included sections that dealt with the adverse health effects of the substances being considered. The health-effects sections would correspond to the Committee's definition of hazard identification.

The legislative history of the Act makes it clear that Congress intended a close coupling between NIOSH's recommendations and OSHA's standards. Nevertheless, relatively few NIOSH criteria documents have led to OSHA standards. This disjunction between the two agencies has stemmed from the difficulty of coordinating two organizations that are physically separated and responsible to different departments. As mentioned earlier, the degree to which OSHA has relied on NIOSH for its scientific expertise has varied. In the early 1970s, OSHA relied heavily on NIOSH for evaluation of health effects; later, OSHA developed its own staff of health scientists and, with considerable help from consultants and contractors, performed its own risk assessments to support agency standard-setting activities.

Because OSHA conducts its own assessments of risk, as well as setting standards, and NIOSH does risk assessments and recommends standards, the relation of NIOSH and OSHA as it has existed since 1976 represents, in some sense, duplication, rather than true extra-agency separation. The earlier relation between the two agencies is, however, an example of extra-agency separation. This section focuses on NIOSH's production of criteria documents during both phases and reflects procedures used throughout the 1970s.

Agenda and Procedures

In the past, NIOSH had an elaborate procedure for setting priorities, which included soliciting nominations of candidate substances from OSHA and the public. In practice, however, before 1976, NIOSH's criteria document agenda was set by agency personnel and the Director, on the basis of their views of the seriousness of various occupational hazards and the number of workers exposed to such hazards. OSHA played little or no role in the selection process, and NIOSH's agenda for documents therefore did not reflect or greatly influence OSHA's regulatory agenda. One cause of this lack of correlation between the two schedules was their physical and organizational separation. In the late 1970s, NIOSH did receive communications from OSHA that led NIOSH to begin production of process- and industry-oriented criteria documents. Table III-5 lists criteria documents transmitted to OSHA.

Methods and Use of Guidelines

Preparation of a criteria document involved a preliminary review of literature and the identification of gaps in the relevant knowledge. This gap analysis was fed into NIOSH's research planning and led to research directed at filling the gaps. Brief studies could be completed in time for their results to be incorporated into the document. Others would continue after the document was completed and sometimes resulted in revision or updating. The literature review and preparation of a draft document were commonly performed by an external contractor under the supervision of NIOSH personnel. Because NIOSH does not have written guidelines for risk assessment, whether personnel preparing the documents used similar approaches to evaluate data and reach conclusions regarding risks is unclear. NIOSH's failure to develop risk assessment guidelines has helped to obscure the distinction between scientific and policy judgments in the risk assessment process. Although the rationale for separating NIOSH from OSHA has been to allow an independent scientific evaluation without the consideration of economic implications that is necessary in OSHA rule-making activities, the effectiveness of this institutional separation in eliminating the effects of such risk management considerations on the conduct of risk assessment by NIOSH is difficult to determine.

Peer Review

The initial review of a draft criteria document was typically performed by NIOSH staff in the same division of the agency that produced the document. The division draft was then submitted to other NIOSH divisions for review. This was followed by a review performed by knowledgeable experts from industry, labor organizations,

TABLE III-5 NIOSH Criteria Documents Sent to
OSHA by May 1982

Substance or Subject	Transmitted to OSHA	
Acetylene	1976	
Acrylamide	1976	
Acrylonitrile	1977	
Alkanes	1977	
Allyl chloride	1976	
Ammonia	1974	
Antimony	1978	
Arsenic, inorganic	1974,	1975
Asbestos	1972,	1976
Asphalt fumes	1977	
Benzene	1974,	1977
Benzoyl peroxide	1977	
Benzyl chloride	1978	
Beryllium	1972,	1977
Boron trifluoride	1976	
Cadmium	1976	
Carbaryl	1976	
Carbon black	1978	
Carbon dioxide	1976	
Carbon disulfide	1977	
Carbon monoxide	1972	
Carbon tetrachloride	1975,	1976
Chlorine	1976	
Chloroform	1974,	1976
Chlorophene	1977	
Chromic acid	1973	
Chromium (VI)	1975	
Coal-gasification plants	1978	
Coal-liquefaction (Vols. I and II)	1981	
Coal-tar products	1977	
Cobalt	1981	
Coke-oven emission	1973	
Confined spaces (as workplaces)	1980	
Cotton dust	1974	
Cresol	1978	
Cyanide, hydrogen, and cyanide salts	1976	
Decomposition products of fluorocarbon	1977	
Dibromochloropropane	1977	
Diisocyanates	1978	
Dinitro-o-cresol	1978	
Dioxane	1977	
Emergency egress from elevated work stations	1975	
Epichlorohydrin	1976	
Ethylene dibromide	1977	
Fibrous glass	1977	
Fluorides, inorganic	1975	
Formaldehyde	1976	
Furfuryl alcohol	1979	
Glycidyl ethers	1978	
Hot environments	1972	
Hydrazines	1978	

TABLE III-5   (Continued)

Substance or Subject	Transmitted to OSHA
Hydrogen fluoride	1976
Hydrogen sulfide	1977
Hydroquinone	1978
Identification system for occupationally hazardous materials	1974
Isopropyl alcohol	1976
Kepones	1976
Ketones	1978
Lead, inorganic	1973, 1977
Logging--from felling to first haul	1976
Malathion	1976
Mercury, inorganic	1973
Methyl alcohol	1976
Methylene chloride	1976
Methyl parathion	1976
Nickel, inorganic and compounds	1977
Nitric acid	1976
Nitriles	1978
Nitrogen oxides	1976
Nitroglycerin--ethylene glycol dinitrate	1978
Noise	1972
Organotin compounds	1976
Parathion	1976
Pesticide manufacturing and formulation	1978
Phenol	1976
Phosgene	1976
Polychlorinated biphenyls	1977
Refined petroleum solvent	1977
Silica, crystalline	1974
Sodium hydroxide	1975
Sulfur dioxide	1974, 1977
Sulfuric acid	1974
1,1,2,2-Tetrachloroethane	1976
Tetrachloroethylene	1976
Thiols: n-alkane mono-, cyclohexane, and benzene	1978
Toluene	1973
Toluene diisocyanate	1973, 1978
o-Toluidine	1978
1,1,1-Trichloroethane	1976
Tungsten and cemented tungsten carbide	1977
Ultraviolet radiation	1972
Vanadium	1977
Vinyl acetate	1978
Vinyl chloride	1974
Vinyl halides	1978
Waste anesthetic gases and vapors	1977
Xylene	1975
Zinc oxide	1975

and universities. In addition, other appropriate government agencies, professional associations, and trade
organizations were invited to review the document. After
these various reviews were complete and changes were made
as deemed appropriate by division staff, the document was
forwarded to the Director of NIOSH.

Several shortcomings of NIOSH criteria documents were
cited in a recent review of the program funded by the
agency: the lack of field experience of criteria document
managers, the lack of critical analysis of data, and the
alleged disregard of reviewers' comments. The latter
claim highlights the importance of procedures that ensure
that reviewers' comments are adequately addressed. The
lack of critical analysis of data has been attributed at
least in part to the facts that the documents were often
developed by outside contractors and that NIOSH had little
control over the personnel assigned to the contract staff.

COMMITTEES OF THE NATIONAL RESEARCH COUNCIL

The National Research Council (NRC) is the operating unit
for the National Academy of Sciences' advisory function.
As part of this advisory function, NRC has been called on
by a number of regulatory agencies to perform risk assessments. Regulatory agencies request assessments by NRC for
several reasons, including statutory requirements that
particular agencies or programs consult with NRC, inade-
quacy of agency staff to perform the assessments (as in
the case of the FDA request for a review of pre-1962
prescription drugs), and such political objectives as a
desire for outside scientific support of an anticipated
agency action or a desire to defuse or postpone controversy. Agencies remain free to accept or reject the
analyses and conclusions included in NRC reports. NRC
risk assessment reports are usually not sufficient by
themselves to dictate specific regulatory action, and a
separate assessment is usually conducted by the agency,
even if in only the most perfunctory fashion.

NRC has done risk assessments for several agencies
with jurisdiction over carcinogenic chemicals. However,
NRC is in no real sense a centralized risk assessment
body and is a very imperfect model for recent proposals
to create such a body. First, most of the evaluative
work of the NRC is actually performed by individual
committees created on an ad hoc basis for each study.
Thus, NRC is not a single risk assessment body, but

rather an umbrella for the work of many diverse, if out-
wardly similar, committees. Second, each ad hoc committee
generally reports to a single agency and does not perform
assessments for several bodies at once. The committees
of NRC have been included in our survey as examples of ad
hoc risk assessment groups that are entirely separate from
government regulators. Table III-6 is a partial list of
NRC reports (published since 1977) that examined the carcinogenic risks associated with exposure to particular
chemicals.

Agenda and Procedures

Committee members are appointed on the strength of their
professional qualifications; they may come from universities, industry, government, or another sector of society, but they do not serve as representatives of any
agency, group, or institution unless they are specifically so designated on appointment. Occasionally when,
by virtue of special expertise or for other reasons, persons affiliated with interested parties are placed on
committees, every effort is made to achieve a balance of
interests. In any case, all committee members are asked
to complete a statement, "On Potential Sources of Bias,"
which includes information on sources of personal income,
sources of research support, and more subtle forms of
personal bias, including values held that may influence a
member's judgment. The membership of every committee that
will formulate a position, take an action, or prepare a
report is reviewed by NRC staff and must be approved by
the Chairman of NRC. The work of the committees is facil-
itated by professional and support staff employed by NRC.
   The conduct of a study varies with its nature and
objective, the time permitted to complete it, its political sensitivity, and the personalities involved. In general, committees have considerable latitude in carrying
out their responsibilities and may hold public meetings
and schedule technical conferences to collect pertinent
information. Committees typically meet three to six
times a year. Meetings are concerned with planning,
discussions of issues and drafts of reports, and, later,
the development of final conclusions and recommendations.
Although a committee has much freedom in planning and
executing its study and reaching its conclusions, several
restrictions include the obvious necessity to respond to
the charge stipulated in the contract, time and budgetary

TABLE III-6   Some NRC Reports Dealing with
Carcinogenic Chemicals (1977-1982)

Report	Parent Unit[a]	Year
An Assessment of Mercury in the Environment	CPSMR	1977
An Evaluation of the Carcino-genicity of Chlordane and Heptachlor	CLS	1977
Drinking Water and Health	CLS	1977
Arsenic	CLS	1977
Nitrates	CPSMR	1978
Saccharin--Technical Assessment of Risks and Benefits	CLS	1978
Polychlorinated Biphenyls	CPSMR	1979
Drinking Water and Health, Vol. III	CLS	1980
The Alkyl Benzenes	CLS	1980
Formaldehyde--An Assessment of Its Health Effects	CLS	1980
Regulating Pesticides	CPSMR	1980
Aromatic Amines: An Assessment of the Biological and Environmental Effects	CLS	1981
Formaldehyde and Other Aldehydes	CLS	1981
The Health Effects of Nitrate, Nitrite, and N-Nitroso Compounds	CLS	1981
Indoor Pollutants	CLS	1981
Selected Aliphatic Amines and Related Compounds: An Assessment of the Biological and Environmental Effects	CLS	1981
Alternatives to the Current Use of Nitrite in Foods	CLS	1982
An Assessment of the Health Risks of Seven Pesticides for Termite Control	CLS	1982
Diet, Nutrition, and Cancer	CLS	1982
Drinking Water and Health, Vol. IV	CLS	1982
Quality Criteria for Water Reuse	CLS	1982
Possible Long-Term Health Effects of Short-Term Exposure to Chemical Agents, Vol. 1--Anticholinesterases and Anticholinergics	CLS	1982

[a]CPSMR = Commission on Physical Sciences, Mathematics,
and Resources; CLS = Commission on Life Sciences.

limitations, and the necessity for a central NRC-monitored review of the final report.

In addition to providing scientific analyses on which policy or regulatory decisions can be based, NRC reports sometimes make specific recommendations for changes in government policy.

Methods and Use of Guidelines

NRC risk assessments are not easily classified or characterized. Because different committees prepare risk-related reports and NRC does not have any guidelines on the conduct of risk assessments for the committees to follow, approaches and final products show pronounced variations. The absence of guidelines, coupled with the occasional practice of not including a clear explanation of how conclusions concerning risk were reached or of the assumptions used in the quantitation of risk, has led to a blurring of the distinction between scientific and policy judgments made in the assessment of risks. The lack of guidelines has also led to inconsistencies in approach and final decisions among committees. However, the absence of specific guidance for interpreting data and for choosing methods of dose-response assessment or risk characterization is probably to be expected, inasmuch as NRC committees consist of scientific experts whose independent judgments are being sought. Probably only guidelines that are extremely flexible could be adopted by NRC. A subject of much discussion over the last several years has been the value of including quantitative assessments (in our terms, dose-response assessments or, if exposure data are incorporated, risk characterizations) in reports. The trend in recent years has been to include some form of a quantitative risk estimate.

Peer Review

Every report from the NRC is reviewed by a group other than the authors. The process of reviewing is overseen by the Report Review Committee. The reports likely to receive reviews coordinated by that Committee are those judged to have significant policy implications and likely to be controversial; most reports that address risk-related questions would be in this category. (The Report Review Committee also coordinates the review of noncontro-

versial reports on an ad hoc basis to monitor the overall
quality of NRC reports.) A report not receiving such a
review is reviewed under the auspices of its parent commission, independent office, or board. Report Review
Committee review entails submission of a draft report to
a set of reviewers selected in a cooperative process by
the the parent body and the Report Review Committee.
These reviewers are invited to comment on technical
adequacy and accuracy (the expertness of the authors), on
clarity and appropriateness of presentation, on response
to charge, on cogency of recommendations with respect to
data presented, and on degree of objectivity and freedom
from bias. The committee and staff respond to reviewers'
criticisms and suggestions, and the responses are examined by a monitor, usually a member of the Report Review
Committee, to determine their appropriateness. Thus, a
person outside the unit that prepared the report decides
whether adequate consideration has been given to reviewers' comments. In cases of persistent and severe
disagreement between reviewers and authors, the matter
may be referred to the NRC chairman for resolution.

    Like the regulatory agencies, NRC has been the subject
of controversy in recent years. Some NRC committees have
been accused of bias related to their judgments on the
risks associated with the substances they are studying.
The absence of a member from a discipline that is important for a balanced assessment of risk can also weaken
the credibility of an NRC report. For example, an internal NRC study (1981) stated that, in a small sample of
risk-related studies completed before 1979, such disciplines as epidemiology were often not represented on the
rosters of committees whose subjects appeared to warrant
such knowledge.

FDA'S DRUG EVALUATION PANELS

Under the Federal Food, Drug, and Cosmetic Act, FDA
regulates the marketing of all medicines for human
use--prescription pharmaceuticals, over-the-counter
drugs, and biologic products, which are also subject to
the 1902 Biologics Act. In its efforts to ensure the
safety and effectiveness of drugs in these three classes,
FDA has relied heavily on advisory panels composed
primarily of scientists from academic medicine. Two
major programs illustrate the important role of such
independent expert panels in agency assessments of human

drugs: the Drug Efficacy Study, a review of the effectiveness of pre-1962 prescription drugs undertaken by NRC in 1966; and the over-the-counter Drug Review, in which advisory panels established directly by FDA have evaluated the effectiveness and safety of ingredients of such drugs.

Both the NRC review and the FDA-directed review enabled FDA to undertake systematic studies of product performance that would have overwhelmed the agency's own resources and personnel. The two reviews differed in a number of respects that may shed some light on optimal structures and procedures for scientific panels.

NRC Review

The 1962 Kefauver-Harris Amendments to the Federal Food, Drug, and Cosmetic Act required that all new drugs be proved effective, as well as safe, and obliged FDA, after a 2-year grace period, to require proof of efficacy of all pre-1962 drugs. In discharging this obligation for prescription drugs, the agency turned to NRC to establish some 30 panels of six to eight experts in pharmaceutical therapy; each panel was responsible for a class of drugs.

The panels evaluated the data supplied to them by FDA and manufacturers and rated the drugs as effective, probably effective, possibly effective, ineffective, ineffective as a fixed combination, or inferior to other better or safer therapies for the same indications. Their main function was thus to assess therapeutic efficacy, not risk to patient health (except indirectly); all the drugs reviewed had been judged to be safe before original FDA approval. Nevertheless, the panels included comments on the safety of individual drugs, particularly those whose effectiveness was in doubt. An informal NRC coordinating group attempted to review each panel's ratings before forwarding them to FDA, in the hope of ensuring some consistency. In practice, however, the panel's verdicts reached FDA largely unreviewed.

The clinical and other data on which the panels relied came from FDA files, the medical and scientific literature, and the manufacturers of the drugs. The panels neither performed nor ordered any new research, although their assessments often identified subjects on which further studies were needed. The panels met and worked privately; apart from being invited to submit supporting data, manufacturers had no opportunity to participate in the panels' deliberations, nor did representatives of consumers or FDA staff.

To reconstruct precisely how the panels worked or to determine what criteria for evaluation each followed is difficult. The predetermined categories in which they were to rate drugs produced apparent homogeneity in their results, but did not sharply confine or direct their analyses. Evidently, wide variations occurred among the panels. The panels' assessments were reported to FDA largely as statements of conclusions; many of the reports were only one or two paragraphs long. Explanations for the ratings typically took the form of bare references to published studies or invocations of the informed judgment of the panelists. In short, the panels provided verdicts, rather than documented evaluations.

The weight to be given the panels' assessments was not squarely addressed when FDA contracted for NRC assistance. Apparently, it was understood that FDA remained free to accept or reject a panel's judgment, but it must have expected to accept most of the panels' assessments when it contracted with NRC. The agency's primary goal was to spare its own scientific staff the enormous burden of evaluating the effectiveness of thousands of pre-1962 drugs. In practice, FDA has accorded substantial weight to the assessments provided by the NRC panels, usually accepting the rating provided and initiating appropriate regulatory action. A rating of less than "effective" led to notification of a drug manufacturer that more data were needed to support a claim of effectiveness; later (often years later), if data were still considered inadequate, the agency took steps to remove the drug from the market. Some of the agency's efforts provoked protracted litigation and administrative hearings. However, pharmaceutical manufacturers have acceded to the panels' judgments in the majority of instances, occasionally by withdrawing products from the market, more frequently by eliminating claims for which supporting evidence was lacking, and sometimes by sponsoring new clinical research. One important determinant of the acceptance of panel assessments was the commercial importance of the product or claim at issue. When a panel rating and ultimate FDA judgment jeopardized the continued marketing of an important product, the manufacturer often insisted on its full legal rights in the course of combating FDA's efforts at implementation.

FDA-Directed Drug Panels

The NRC review of pre-1962 drugs did not address the marketing status of most over-the-counter drugs. In 1972,
FDA launched a second comprehensive review, this time on
both the effectiveness and the safety of all active ingredients in over-the-counter drugs. At the outset of this
review, FDA chartered 17 advisory committees representing
therapeutic groupings. These 17 panels met a total of 522
times over a 9-year period; they reviewed 722 active
ingredients for over 1,400 indications and submitted over
75 reports on different therapeutic categories, e.g.,
internal analgesics, antimicrobials, and vaginal
contraceptives.

The central function of these review panels was to
report and explain their assessments of the safety and
effectiveness of the ingredients used in over-the-counter
drugs. These reports were to set forth not only the
panels' judgments rating each ingredient (as generally
recognized as safe and effective, as unsafe or ineffective, or as requiring additional study), but also supporting documentation and rationale. The panel reports
became treatises on the various therapeutic categories,
some well over 1,000 pages long. The recommendation
segments of the reports were considerably shorter.

FDA intended from the outset to rely heavily on the
panels' assessments and thus insisted that they produce
thoroughly documented findings. In addition, the panels
were required to meet in public and to adhere to other
requirements of the Federal Advisory Committee Act.
Together, these obligations prolonged the panels' deliberations. Although the Antacid Panel completed its report
in less than a year, more complex categories, containing
more ingredients, occupied panels for several years,
during which they may have met once a month.

The responsibility of producing a fully documented
report required the panels to rely on FDA staff to
assemble information, handle administrative and steno-
graphic responsibilities, and often do much of the
drafting. Thus, the sharp separation that existed
between FDA's Bureau of Drugs and the NRC panels never
characterized its relation with the over-the-counter
panels. However, because discussions of draft reports
were held in public meetings and panel members reached
their judgments in these meetings, the fact that the
final text and judgments represented their views, rather
than those of agency staff, was clear. The assessments

of the panels generally have commanded considerable acceptance, because they were reached through public debate
and were thoroughly documented.

At the outset of the review, FDA forecast that it would
implement most of the panels' assessments. The agency
has released the panels' recommendations in the form of
notices of proposed rule-making, which are published in
the Federal Register as the first step in translating
them into regulations. The Bureau of Drugs has expressly
reserved the privilege of disagreeing with a panel's findings either immediately or in a tentative final monograph,
and it has sometimes done so. These occasions have been
few, but usually controversial; and sometimes the Bureau
has retreated from its initial disagreement. No manufacturer has been successful in overturning, administratively
or in court, a panel judgment in which the Bureau of
Drugs concurred.

Perhaps an even better measure of the credence given
the panels' assessments is the high degree of voluntary
compliance displayed by manufacturers. They have aban-
doned, albeit often reluctantly, most of the ingredients
whose effectiveness the panels have doubted. Almost
without exception, they have acceded to the panels'
safety judgments. Similarly, they have generally accepted
the panels' recommendations for changes in labeling.
This remarkable commercial deference to scientific judgment has several explanations, in addition to the credibility of the panels. The slow pace of the review permitted manufacturers to make changes in their formulas or
labeling without serious market disruption. The procedures of the panels themselves afforded opportunities for
manufacturers to submit information and make arguments
before a judgment was rendered. Perhaps as important,
the panels' assessments, thus far, have not often jeopardized the continued marketing of major products or whole
classes of drugs. If that occurs, it is likely that the
panels' findings will encounter more determined
opposition.

NATIONAL TOXICOLOGY PROGRAM PANEL ON FORMALDEHYDE

The National Toxicology Program (NTP) was established in
1978 by the Secretary of the Department of Health and
Human Services to coordinate all toxicity testing of
chemicals in the Department and to facilitate communication between the research and regulatory agencies. NTP

embraces the relevant toxicity testing activities of the
National Cancer Institute, National Institute of Environmental Health Sciences, FDA (and its National Center for
Toxicological Research), and the Centers for Disease
Control. OSHA, EPA, and CPSC also participate in NTP. A
major advisory group for NTP is its Executive Committee,
which is made up of the heads of the agencies listed
above, as well as the Director of the National Institutes
of Health and the Assistant Secretary for Health. NTP
thus serves as a vehicle for cooperation among the four
regulatory agencies--FDA, EPA, OSHA, and CPSC--especially
in recommending candidate substances for testing. At
least one agency has also called on NTP to review risk
assessments: the FDA has on two occasions asked another
NTP advisory group--the Board of Scientific Counselors--
to review the carcinogenicity data and the agency's analysis of those data on two color additives being considered
for agency approval. In addition, NTP has served on one
occasion as a structure through which a risk assessment
of interest to all four regulatory agencies was performed.

In April 1980, CPSC (in cooperation with the Interagency Regulatory Liaison Group) requested that the NTP
help to form an interagency panel on formaldehyde to
review the carcinogenicity data on this chemical. The
Panel consisted of 16 government scientists, most of whom
were experts in toxicology, pharmacology, and epidemiology. Three of the IRLG agencies--EPA, FDA, and OSHA--
also supplied scientists as members. Although no employee
of CPSC was an official Panel member, a liaison representative of the agency attended all meetings and contributed
to portions of the final report. In addition, CPSC personnel assisted the Panel by preparing bibliographies and
handling arrangements.

The Panel on Formaldehyde thus serves as an example of
a centralized assessment body that, although placed
outside the agencies, maintained some association with
the scientific staffs of each. The decision to confine
the membership to government scientists was driven, in
part, by a desire to avoid delays associated with compliance with the Federal Advisory Committee Act's requirements for establishing outside committees. The Panel's
creation was viewed as an experiment in interagency
coordination.

The Panel met three times. It generally deliberated
in private, and its meetings were not announced. The
Panel did consult with Chemical Industry Institute of
Toxicology scientists who were responsible for designing

and conducting the carcinogenicity study being evaluated,
and it permitted both oral and written statements from
the Formaldehyde Institute, a trade association of users
and manufacturers. Although the Panel reported its findings somewhat later than initially forecast by CPSC, the
time required was a relatively brief 6-7 months. One
unanticipated delay resulted from the necessity for a
second review of the pathology slides from the major
study being evaluated. The report stated that evaluation
of the findings on carcinogenic effect and other related
data convinced the Panel members that formaldehyde is an
animal carcinogen when inhaled. This finding has been
supported by many other scientists, and the Panel's report
has since been published in a peer-reviewed scientific
journal. The Panel also concluded that none of the available epidemiologic studies negated the inference that
formaldehyde posed a cancer risk for humans. It did not
attempt to estimate the risk of cancer for any exposed
segment of the population. It did include, however, a
quantitative dose-response assessment.

The NTP Panel's formation and performance demonstrate
that such ad hoc collaboration is manageable and can
function well. Despite the quality of its report and its
timely production, however, the NTP Panel's deliberations
and report have not yielded any regulatory efficiencies.
In early 1982, CPSC banned further use of urea-formal-
dehyde foam insulation, in part on the basis of the
Panel's report, as well as the agency's own risk assessments of formaldehyde's acute and chronic effects. In
contrast, EPA has declined to initiate regulation of
formaldehyde in response to the Panel's assessment. The
Agency declined to act under Section 4(f) of the Toxic
Substances Control Act, noting that the animal data available on carcinogenicity did not constitute a "reasonable
basis to conclude that [formaldehyde] presents or will
present a significant risk of serious or widespread harm
to human beings from cancer. . . ." However, because the
Agency's posture is equivocal and not clearly documented,
the degree to which it relied on the Panel's assessment
in reaching the conclusion is unclear.

Neither of the other two agencies followed CPSC's
lead. OSHA declined to issue an emergency standard for
worker exposure to formaldehyde, concluding that it poses
no imminent hazard; and it recently announced that it was
unable to proceed to establish a permanent standard,
because the evidence of animal carcinogenicity did not

reveal what, if any, risk exposed workers might confront. These decisions were also based on OSHA's own assessment of risks, but the degree to which OSHA relied on the Panel's assessment for the agency's hazard identification step is unclear. Both EPA and OSHA are continuing to collect data on formaldehyde, but no regulatory action appears likely in the near future. FDA has not acted, because the potential formaldehyde exposures from agency-regulated products were judged to be very low.

The contrasting regulatory outcomes should not be interpreted as indicative that the Panel on Formaldehyde failed in its mission. Although the four agencies planned to consider its report carefully, the Panel's findings were not expected to be binding. Each agency remained free not only to fashion its own regulatory response on formaldehyde, but to qualify, or to dissent from, the Panel's determination of carcinogenicity and estimate of risk. Factors other than the Panel report's validity and utility are more likely explanations for the divergent agency responses. First, the Panel's report was sub-mitted shortly before the 1980 national election, whose outcome forecast fundamental shifts in regulatory policy at EPA and OSHA. Second, the agencies confront exposures to formaldehyde that differ widely in character and inten-sity, yielding important differences in potential risk. Finally, the statutory criteria governing their decisions could plausibly lead them to accord different weights to the Panel's findings. OSHA, for example, had to decide whether formaldehyde posed a risk sufficient to justify emergency protective measures despite any costs of immediate action.

EPA'S USE OF SCIENTIFIC REVIEW PANELS

The EPA has had considerable experience with independent scientific panels, but they have served the Agency differ-ently from the risk assessment panels discussed in the preceding section. EPA's panels typically have reviewed the work of Agency scientists and analysts, rather than perform their own risk assessments. Also, most panels serving EPA are mandated by Congress and play legally prescribed roles in the Agency's decision-making process. We examined two such panels: EPA's Scientific Advisory Panel and the Subcommittee on Airborne Carcinogens (a unit of EPA's Science Advisory Board).

EPA's Scientific Advisory Panel (SAP)

The Scientific Advisory Panel was established by Congress
in the 1975 Federal Insecticide, Fungicide, and Rodenticide Act to review EPA's evaluations of the environmental
and health risks posed by specific pesticide uses. Broadly speaking, the Panel reviews risk assessments prepared
by EPA's Office of Pesticide Programs to support contemplated regulatory actions against hazardous pesticides.
It also reviews the proposed and final forms of such
actions. Consultation was initially required only when
the Agency contemplated suspending or canceling a pesticide's registration or issuing general regulations
governing pesticide registration. Cancellations and
general pesticide regulations must be submitted to the
Panel for review before they take effect. Suspensions of
registration do not require prior review, but EPA must
submit the underlying studies for review promptly after
any suspension action. EPA must also submit for peer
review the "design, protocols, and conduct of major scientific studies" conducted under the pesticide act. The
following description reflects activities undertaken
before September 1981.*

The Panel normally consists of seven members selected
by the EPA Administrator from among six persons nominated
by the National Institutes of Health and six nominated by
the National Science Foundation. Until its last meeting
in June 1981, the Panel generally met once a month.
Topics covered during 1980 and 1981 are shown in Table
III-7. The Panel does not set its own agenda, although
the chairman may control the sequence and conduct of individual sessions. The risk assessments that the Panel
reviews are selected by the two divisions (Hazard Evaluation and Special Pesticide Review) of the Office of
Pesticide Programs that use its recommendations. Virtu-
ally all the scientific and exposure information available to the Panel is provided by the division whose
assessment is being reviewed, although much of this
information comes originally from the registrant of the
product in question. Panel members necessarily accept
the authenticity of the information provided, although
they sometimes question its quality.

---

*Authorizing legislation expired in September 1981, and
new legislation has not been enacted (as of December
1982).

TABLE III-7 EPA Actions Reviewed by the Scientific
Advisory Panel (1980-1981)

A. Regulations under Section 25(a) of The Federal
   Insecticide, Fungicide, and Rodenticide Act

   1. Final Rulemaking for Registering Pesticides in the
      United States, Subpart E, Hazard Evaluation:
      Wildlife and Aquatic Organisms
   2. Proposed Rulemaking for Registering Pesticides in
      the United States, Subpart L, Hazard Evaluation:
      Nontarget Insects
   3. Proposed and Final Rulemaking for Registering
      Pesticides in the United States, Subpart D,
      Chemistry Requirements: Product Chemistry
   4. Final Rulemaking for Amendment of 40 CFR 162.31 by
      Adding Certain Uses of Eight Active Ingredients as
      Restricted Pesticides
   5. Proposed Rulemaking for Registering Pesticides in
      the United States, Subpart M, Data Requirements
      for Biorational Pesticides
   6. Final Rulemaking for Registering Pesticides in the
      United States, Subpart N, Chemistry Requirements:
      Environmental Fate
   7. Informal Review of Draft Proposed Pesticide
      Registration Guidelines, Subpart K, Exposure Data
      Requirements: Reentry Protection
   8. Review of Proposed Pesticide Registration
      Guidelines, Subpart H, Labeling of Pesticide
      Products
   9. Review of Final Rule on Classification of 11
      Active Ingredients for Restricted Use

B. Cancellations under Section 6(b) of the Federal
   Insecticide, Fungicide, and Rodenticide Act

   1. Dimethoate
   2. Diallate
   3. Lindane
   4. Strychnine
   5. Ethylene dibromide
   6. Oxyfluorfen (Goal 2E)
   7. Wood preservatives, pentachlorophenol, creosote,
      arsenicals

Meetings are open to the public, and interested parties are generally encouraged to make presentations. These meetings sometimes focus on risk management issues, rather than on the health and environmental assessments submitted to the Panel, in part because participants making presentations are not confined to addressing scientific aspects of the Agency's risk assessments. Equally important in the consideration of nonscientific issues has been Congress's decision not to restrict the Panel to a strictly scientific review of the Agency's risk assessments. (The Panel's mandated review responsibilities extend to contemplated EPA actions that combine both risk assessment and regulatory policy elements.) Although the rationale for the Panel's creation was to introduce independent scientific review into EPA's deliberations, the mechanism chosen has routinely resulted in the Panel's commenting on the Agency's choice of regulatory options. The Agency has sought to anticipate the Panel's tendency to stray from the scientific issues before it and has attempted to frame specific questions on which comments are requested.

The participation of the Panel probably has improved the quality of EPA analyses and added to their credibility among both environmental and industry groups. However, expectations of some EPA critics that it would repudiate the Agency's scientific analyses have not been realized. Over the last 5 years, the Panel has agreed with most Agency risk assessments brought before it. There have been some notable exceptions, such as the Panel's disagreement with the Agency's handling of 2,4,5-T. The endorsement of most Agency assessments and Agency actions based on those assessments by the Panel have been extremely helpful in improving Agency credibility and rendered its actions less vulnerable to challenge in administrative or judicial hearings, as with the Panel's support of EPA action on wood preservatives. The Panel's success can be traced to several causes: its public deliberations, which may have made it difficult for EPA to ignore its comments; its continuity (until its authorizing legislation expired), which permitted it to understand EPA's approaches and simultaneously strengthened its influence with EPA staff; and the scientific distinction of individual Panel members.

In the case of EPA's decision to suspend use of 2,4,5-T and Silvex (its companion product) for some applications and to hold wide-ranging hearings on other applications, the Panel declined, after 3 days of public meetings, to support the Agency's proposed proceedings.

The Panel believed that additional data, including results
of further tests for carcinogenicity and reproductive toxicity and of more complete monitoring for residues, were
required before a hearing could be held profitably.
Because EPA had not asked the Panel to approve the hold-
ing of a hearing and believed that it would be more
efficient to deal with all uses of 2,4,5-T at one time,
the Agency persisted and announced a hearing on the risks
and benefits of 2,4,5-T, which began in March 1980. This
difference, coupled with congressional displeasure with
EPA's original suspension of 2,4,5-T and Silvex, led ultimately to the 1980 statutory amendment mandating that the
Scientific Advisory Panel review the studies that underlie
suspension decisions.

EPA's Subcommittee on Airborne Carcinogens

The Subcommittee on Airborne Carcinogens, a part of EPA's
Science Advisory Board, was not mandated by statute. It
was created in 1980 at the request of the Assistant
Administrator for Air, Noise, and Radiation to review the
assessments that the Agency is statutorily required to
submit for Board review. Members of this Subcommittee
were appointed by the Administrator; however, it no longer
exists, having recently been merged with the Environmental Health Committee of the Science Advisory Board.
    The Subcommittee reviewed six pairs of draft documents
that included hazard identification and dose-response
assessments produced by the Carcinogen Assessment Group
and exposure assessments produced by private contractors
for EPA's Office of Air Quality Planning and Standards.
The chemicals evaluated in those documents were trichloro-
ethylene, perchloroethylene, methylene chloride, methyl
chloroform, acrylonitrile, and toluene. Subcommittee
members reviewing these documents included a biochemist,
a biostatistician, a pathologist, an engineer, an oncolo-
gist, a toxicologist, and a meteorologist. Five members
were affiliated with universities and one with a research
consulting organization; the seventh was a private consultant.
    In accordance with the Federal Advisory Committee Act,
the Subcommittee's review was held in public and announced
in the Federal Register, and interested members of the
public were invited to make oral and written presentations. Several such presentations were made, primarily
by representatives of industries that would be affected

by EPA regulation of the substances under discussion.
EPA and contractor personnel also attended the review and
participated actively, briefing the Subcommittee on the
contents of documents, answering members' questions, and
defending their work against criticism.

The Subcommittee did not write a report after its
review, and the absence of a summary report has led to
some confusion regarding the nature of its criticisms.
Review of the transcript of its second meeting (September
5, 1980) and discussions with various participants in that
review meeting have revealed several general criticisms
of the Carcinogen Assessment Group's risk assessments.
One was that the documents provided to the Subcommittee
were not sufficiently detailed; i.e., they did not provide enough scientific information from the various
studies cited to permit the Subcommittee to make an independent assessment of the quality and validity of the
studies. Another criticism raised by the Subcommittee
was that the conclusions drawn did not reflect the
quality of the data on which the risk assessments were
based. Some Subcommittee members asserted that such
considerations may, in fact, be precluded by rigid
adherence to the Agency's guidelines for risk assessment.

Other criticisms focused on specific issues, including
the validity of basing a conclusion of carcinogenicity on
an increase in mouse liver tumors, the importance of
contaminants in the test chemicals, and the wisdom of
using a single model for extrapolating from high to low
doses. The Subcommittee viewed these issues as primarily
scientific, whereas Agency staff considered them, although
resting on scientific principles, as resolvable through
the choice of conservative policy options--a choice
embodied in the Agency's guidelines. These differences
between the Subcommittee and Agency staff emphasize the
conclusion set forth in Chapter I that many components of
risk assessment lack a firm scientific answer and require
a judgment to be made. In some cases, such judgments may
be informed by scientific arguments, but may ultimately
rest on policy preferences. The difficulties in communication between the Agency and the Subcommittee also under-
score the importance of explicit risk assessments and
written reviews.

The differences reported above have not yet been fully
resolved. The Agency's experience with the Subcommittee
highlights some difficulties in using a review body that
has not had sufficient time to develop a working approach
to its task. It also emphasizes the importance of ex-

plaining Agency risk assessment procedures, including the adherence to specific guidelines, to review panels. Concerns similar to those of the Subcommittee have been expressed by members of the Environmental Health Committee, which replaced it, and Agency staff are currently considering changes in the risk assessment procedures embodied in their guidelines.

PROPOSED CHANGES IN ORGANIZATIONAL ARRANGEMENTS
FOR RISK ASSESSMENT

Proposals to reform the organizational arrangements for risk assessment have been advanced to reduce perceived shortcomings in agency practices. The criticisms to which these proposals respond may be summarized as follows:

* Bias. Critics of agency performance suggest that decision-makers approach risk assessment with attitudes about regulation that preclude objectivity. Regulators, for example, may skew their assessment of risks associated with a particular substance to support a preference to regulate or not to regulate that substance.

* Exaggeration. This criticism is closely related to the first. The suggestion is that regulatory agencies, accustomed to operating in an adversary mode and expecting their judgments to be challenged in administrative hearings or in court, typically overstate the risks associated with hazards that they decide to regulate or understate the risks associated with hazards that they decide not to regulate. The instinct to support a position with every available argument may distort interpretations of scientific data, choice of extrapolation procedures, and assumptions about human exposure. The critical role of legal staff in preparing agency documents is thought to foster the adversarial style.

* Poor Public Understanding. If risks are misdescribed, it follows that public perception of the risks will be inaccurate. In addition, because agency announcements of regulatory actions typically stress the ultimate risk management strategy, such as the banning of saccharin, and do not explain why a particular action is being taken, the public is led to infer the degree of risk from the action proposed or from the decision not to act. However, an agency's ultimate decision may be dictated by statutory language or regulatory policies that emphasize considerations other than degree of risk.

* <u>Poor-Quality Personnel</u>. This argument is straightforward, if unflattering. It is that regulatory agencies cannot attract or retain adequate numbers of highly qualified scientists to perform risk assessments. Many of their personnel are removed from active research by time and distance and are unfamiliar with the latest developments in their fields.

* <u>Inconsistency</u>. This criticism supports proposals for centralization of risk assessment. To the extent that separation is a prerequisite to centralization, this criticism would also support institutional separation. The suggestion is simply that agencies have applied inconsistent criteria and reached inconsistent results in assessing the risks posed by the same hazards. Such inconsistency is more likely when each agency is responsible for performing its own assessment.

* <u>Redundancy</u>. Starting from the assumption that different regulatory agencies have been, and are likely often to be, concerned with the same hazards, the critics argue that current arrangements force government regulators, affected industries, and interested scientists to deal with litigation on the risks of a given substance several times. Accordingly, a central institution responsible for performing risk assessments for all agencies might yield process efficiencies and reduce costs for all participants.

DESCRIPTION OF PROPOSALS

The central proposals for changes in institutional arrangements for risk assessments developed by the Office of Science and Technology Policy (OSTP) and the American Industrial Health Council (AIHC) and presented in H.R. 638 have sparked much of the current debate and precipitated this study. For several years before, however, dissatisfaction had been expressed with the procedures by which government bodies used scientific data and resolved what purported to be scientific issues. This dissatisfaction led to one of the precursors of the current proposals: the idea of a science court for resolving scientific issues underlying regulatory decisions. That suggestion and other, more recent proposals for procedural and structural reforms are discussed briefly below. The primary objective of this section, however, is to facilitate evaluation of the three main proposals that inspired this study.

Science Court

An important precursor of the OSTP proposal was the
science court concept of Kantrowitz (1975). The science
court was proposed to assist decision-makers with disputed
scientific aspects of a decision. Hence, a basic premise
of the science court is that it is both possible and
desirable to separate the scientific elements of a public-
policy decision from social and political considerations.
The judges of a court were to be impartial, competent
scientists from relevant disciplines who were not involved
in the dispute. These judges would hear testimony from
scientific experts on both sides of the issue, who would
be allowed to cross-examine each other. The rationale
was that scientist advocates are best qualified to present
their own cases and to probe the weaknesses of their
opposition. In the environment created in such a court,
complete objectivity would be neither assumed nor necessary. After hearing all witnesses, the judges would
issue a summary of their opinion of the meaning of the
scientific evidence. Their opinions would deal only with
scientific questions and could not include recommendations for public policy. Many details of a science
court's procedures and operations are, however, unclear.
Even after several years of sometimes heated debate in
the scientific and regulatory communities, the overall
reactions to the concept can be characterized as at best
only lukewarm. Although a genuine science court will
probably not be established, the underlying idea of
separation of scientific issues from social and political
considerations in decision-making has since appeared in
other proposals.
    FDA's creation and use of public boards of inquiry is
the nearest analogue to the science court that has been
put into practice. In 1975, FDA, on its own initiative,
adopted regulations describing a public board of inquiry,
a new kind of decisional body that could substitute for
the traditional trial type of hearing before an administrative law judge if parties to formal disputes before
the agency could agree. A board of inquiry is an ad hoc
panel of three independent scientists, qualified in
relevant disciplines, who hear evidence and arguments and
render a preliminary decision, which may be appealed
(like that of an administrative law judge) to the Commissioner of FDA. The procedure assumes that disputes
that are primarily scientific can be resolved more
accurately, faster, and with greater credibility by an

expert tribunal. FDA's novel procedure has been tried only once, to resolve safety issues concerning aspartame, a new artificial sweetener. This experience yielded, at best, equivocal support for the new procedure. Perhaps because of its novelty, the process took over a year to complete. The parties disagreed at length over the makeup of the board, the objectivity of its members, and the procedures it should follow. The FDA Commissioner ultimately rejected the board's conclusion that aspartame should not be approved and issued an opinion that both questioned the board's scientific rationale and corrected its interpretation of the legal criteria for approval of food additives. Other regulatory disputes, including FDA's refusal to approve the injectable contraceptive, Depo-Provera, are scheduled to be heard by boards of inquiry.

OSTP Proposal

A 1978 report from OSTP gave impetus to emerging proposals for separation and centralization of scientific aspects of risk assessment. The report recommended several steps to ensure consistency in the identification, characterization, and assessment of potential human carcinogens. Two interrelated stages in regulatory decision-making were delineated: Stage I, identification of a substance as a potential human carcinogen, qualitative and quantitative characterization of the risk it poses, and explication of the uncertainties; and Stage II, evaluation of regulatory options and their consequences. This dichotomy closely parallels our own distinction between risk assessment and risk management. The OSTP report recommended that a uniform decision-making framework be used in all agencies and that Stage I and Stage II functions be separated within or outside regulatory agencies while sufficient linkages were maintained to ensure relevance and timeliness. Such organizational experiments as the Carcinogen Assessment Group in EPA were highlighted. The report also suggested that the then-fledgling National Toxicology Program might eventually assume an expanded role in coordinating or overseeing some risk assessments for the regulatory agencies.

H.R. 638 and the AIHC Proposal

The 1978 OSTP report was a broad statement of principles.
Two detailed proposals to create new risk assessment
institutions have since been advanced. Because these
proposals have several features in common, but also
present important contrasts, they are summarized together
(Table III-8).

In February 1980, Representative William Wampler first
introduced legislation (U.S. Congress, 1981c) to establish
a National Science Council. H.R. 638 calls for the creation of a new panel of scientists, entirely independent
of the regulatory agencies, that would decide disputed
scientific issues posed by regulatory initiatives. The
AIHC had previously (1979) advanced a similar proposal to
create an expert science panel that would evaluate the
hazards of chemicals considered for regulation. Both
proposals stress the importance of uniform, consistent
resolution of the scientific questions underlying regulatory decisions. Both espouse the separation of risk
assessment from the design and selection of regulatory
responses, and both would use independent scientific
experts to perform the assessments.

There are some basic differences between the two
proposals. Under H.R. 638, any party could request
referral of scientific issues to the National Science
Council. The AIHC proposal specifies that, although any
party may request a review, only federal agencies or
Congress would have the authority to initiate mandatory
review of scientific questions by the central science
panel. H.R. 638 would apply only in formal adjudications.
The AIHC proposal would apply to any agency proceeding in
which risk assessment was at issue. Because rule-making
is the primary mode for regulating hazardous substances,
the AIHC proposal would apply to more regulatory actions
than would H.R. 638. Under H.R. 638, decisions of the
National Science Council would be binding on regulatory
agencies. In contrast, assessments of the AIHC's science
panel would not bind the agencies, but would carry a
presumption of validity, subject to rebuttal in later
regulatory proceedings.

The risk assessment bodies contemplated by the two
proposals also differ in composition and procedures. The
National Science Council would be a standing body of 15
full-time voting members serving 2-year terms. Individual
chemicals would be assessed initially by advisory panels
made up only of Council members. Each panel would have

TABLE III-8 Comparison of Major Features of H.R. 638
and the AIHC Proposal

H.R. 638	AIHC Proposal
Structure: Single continuing panel separate from agencies; centralized	Single continuing body with rotating members; in the NAS[a]
Membership: 15 full-time members appointed by chairman of NSB[b] from NAS nominees; members to be qualified, distinguished scientists	15 part-time members selected according to NAS procedures; members to represent the best scientists
Scope: Referral by any party of adjudications involving harm to human health from substances considered by CPSC, FDA, USDA,[c] DHHS,[d] OSHA, and EPA	Referral by any party or agency (only latter require mandatory consideration) concerning proposed rules or agency adjudications; all agencies with regulatory jurisdiction would be affected
Functions: Panel could prepare an independent risk assessment; its decision would be binding on the agency	Panel could prepare an independent risk assessment; its findings would be advisory, but would be part of record
Public Participation: Parties to adjudication would be involved	Federal Register notice of referral would solicit submission of data by public
Implementation: Legislation	Legislation

[a]National Academy of Sciences.
[b]National Science Board.
[c]U.S. Department of Agriculture.
[d]Department of Health and Human Services.

at least five voting members. The AIHC science panel
would be established under the umbrella of the National
Academy of Sciences and consist of 15 part-time members
who would serve for terms of 3 years. The panel could
establish working groups, which could be composed largely
of outside experts. These divergent approaches to placement and composition of the panels and terms of members
reflect different expectations about which status would
attract the best scientists and perhaps about the extent
to which the results would be binding. For example, the
AIHC proposal assumes that distinguished academic and
industry scientists would be unwilling to serve on a
full-time basis for any substantial period.

Under H.R. 638, the National Science Council would
decide scientific questions after conducting a formal
"hearing on the record," in which all parties to the
agency proceeding could participate. Under the AIHC
proposal, referral of scientific issues to the panel
would be announced, and the submission of written evidence and arguments would be invited. The less formal
procedures visualized by the AIHC are consistent with its
objective of obtaining nonbinding expert judgments on
scientific issues that underlie decisions.

The two proposals embody different expectations as to
speed of response. H.R. 638 would require the National
Science Council to make a final report to the referring
agency within 90 days of receiving a dispute. The AIHC
proposal, however, imposes no time limits on the panel's
assessment, except that the panel "operate expeditiously
but not precipitously" (Higginson, 1982).

Single-Agency Proposals

H.R. 638 and the AIHC proposal espouse government-wide
reform of the institutional means for risk assessment.
Other notable recommendations for institutional restructuring have been addressed to individual agencies or
agency programs. In 1981, for example, Senator Orrin
Hatch introduced legislation (U.S. Congress, 1981d) to
amend the food-safety provisions of the Federal Food,
Drug, and Cosmetic Act. His bill included a provision
permitting FDA to request, or affected third parties to
demand, assessment of the risks associated with specific
food constituents, with such assessment to be performed
by a panel of scientific experts appointed by the National
Academy of Sciences. The panel's assessment would be

advisory, rather than binding on the agency. Similar
provisions have appeared in other proposals to revise
government regulation of food safety, including a proposal
developed by the Food Safety Council (1979). These proposals appear to share assumptions underlying the AIHC
proposals: that agency risk assessments cannot be assumed
to be objective, thorough, or expert and that an independent review should be available before a final decision
is made. These proposals for independent scientific
panels differ from H.R. 638 in three important ways:
they would apply to one agency or program; they contemplate only an advisory role, rather than a resolving
function, for the scientific panel; and they would apply
to any agency proceeding in which risk assessments were
at issue. The proposals thus can be viewed as agency- or
program-specific illustrations of the AIHC proposal to
create one central scientific panel to serve all agencies.

One such single-agency proposal has been adopted. In
1981, Congress amended the Consumer Product Safety Act
(U.S. Congress, Omnibus Budget Reconciliation Act, 1981a)
to require CPSC to consult with an ad hoc chronic hazards
advisory panel whenever it contemplates rule-making concerning a product believed to pose a risk of cancer, birth
defects, or gene mutation. A panel will consist of seven
members appointed by the Commission from among 21 scientists nominated by the President of the National Academy
of Sciences. Nominees may not be employees of the government or have any financial ties to any manufacturer or
seller of consumer products. Each nominee must have
"demonstrated the ability to critically assess chronic
hazards and risk to human health presented by the exposure of humans to toxic substances or as demonstrated by
the exposure of animals to such substances." The panel's
responsibility is to prepare for the Commission a report
on the substance that the agency is considering regulating. The panel is to review the scientific data and
other information related to the substance and "determine
if any substance in the product is a carcinogen, mutagen,
or teratogen." The panel will also "include in its report
an estimate, if such an estimate is feasible, of the prob-
able harm to human health that will result from exposure
to the substance." The Act requires that a panel submit
its report within 120 days of convening, unless the Commission allows it additional time. A panel's report
"shall contain a complete statement of the basis for its
determination." The Commission must consider the panel's
report and incorporate its evaluation into any advance

notice of proposed rule-making and any final rule. Apparently, the agency is not bound by a panel's determination of carcinogenicity or its estimation of the risk associated with exposure. Although it appears that each panel is to perform its own risk assessment, the statute is silent on the role to be played by agency staff and on the weight that a panel might legitimately accord to analyses prepared by the agency itself. These panels are exempted from the Federal Advisory Committee Act; the exemption presumably means that they are not required to provide advance notice of their meetings or to deliberate in public. A panel may seek information from third parties, but only through CPSC.

CRITICISMS OF PROPOSALS FOR SEPARATION AND CENTRALIZATION

The four federal regulatory agencies have responded skeptically to proposals to separate and centralize the function of assessing the risks of chemicals that are candidates for regulation (U.S. Congress, 1981b). Other observers have also found flaws in the proposals. A central criticism made by those who argue against full organizational separation between risk assessment and regulatory policy-making is that simply separating risk assessment from the regulatory agencies would not separate science from policy. This argument is based on the fact that the risk assessment process requires analytic choices to be made that rest, at least in part, on the policy consideration of whether to be more or less conservative when determining possible public-health risks. A second point is that, although extra-agency separation of risk assessment may help to minimize the influence of risk management considerations on this process, the agency responsible for deciding what exposure to permit or what costs to impose must make what is ultimately a political judgment based on the extent of risk determined in the risk assessment and often on the benefits and costs of regulatory action and its feasibility and political acceptability. For its decision to be politically acceptable and the decision-maker accountable, the agency must have responsibility for each of these components of regulatory decision-making. A third argument against institutional separation is related to the internal process by which agencies reach decisions. It is claimed that this process is unavoidably an iterative one. Different specialists are called on repeatedly for analysis and advice as an agency

identifies and considers new control options in attempting
to reach a decision. Although this description may overstate the fluidity of internal agency deliberations, it
captures something of their ad hoc character. Closely
coupled with this argument is the necessity for agencies
to retain scientific capability so that they can understand what a risk assessment means and how to use it in
developing risk management strategies. Thus, even if
risk assessment were performed outside the agency, a
scientific staff representing many different disciplines
would still be required, to ensure that an assessment
would be interpreted and used correctly.

Other criticisms of proposals for risk assessment by a
centralized panel stress the logistic difficulties of
meshing independent risk assessment activities with the
internal workings of different agencies. Experience
suggests that it will be difficult for any risk assessment body to meet even generous time limits. Thus, agency
decisions will probably be delayed by a requirement to
consult, or refer issues to, such a body. A central
panel also might become overburdened and cause additional
delays. Critics of H.R. 638 and the AIHC proposal challenge the assumption that the regulatory agencies have
reached inconsistent conclusions in evaluating various
chemicals. The recent differences in the regulation of
formaldehyde constitute a rare example of disparate
treatment of the same chemical, and even this disparity
may not betray basic disagreement over the interpretation
of scientific data, as distinct from the degree of risk
that justifies regulation. In the past, the agencies
have often selected different control options or imposed
different exposure limits for a given chemical, but these
disparities have typically reflected differences in exposure (and thus in risk characterization) or differences
in regulatory policy or statutory or administrative
requirements; none of the current proposals addresses
such differences.

CONCLUSIONS

The Committee was asked by the Congress to consider "the
merits of an institutional separation of scientific functions of developing objective risk assessment from the
regulatory process of making public and social policy
decisions and the feasibility of unifying risk assessment
functions." In this chapter, the Committee has addressed

these two issues and a third, related issue: the value
of independent scientific review of agency risk
assessments.

In its review, the Committee was sensitive to a number
of considerations, including the scientific quality and
regulatory relevance of the assessments performed. It
also tried to ascertain how scientific and policy considerations were handled in the performance of risk assessment. To reach its conclusions, in the absence of
accepted criteria for evaluating agency practices and
proposals for change and in view of the sparseness of
relevant empirical data, the Committee has relied on
discussions with other persons knowledgeable and experienced in risk assessment activities, the limited available literature, and especially its own knowledge and
experience in regulatory-agency risk assessments, as well
as its review and analysis of past agency practices.

VALUE OF INSTITUTIONAL SEPARATION

1. Although organizational separation may help to ensure
   that risk management considerations do not influence
   the conduct of risk assessment, the degree of organizational separation that is optimal for individual
   agencies cannot be determined on the basis of the
   Committee's review.

Regulatory programs differ substantially in their
degree of organizational separation. In the cases of
NIOSH assessments that in the early 1970s were adopted by
OSHA and NRC assessments relied on by agencies, the
assessment function has been outside the regulatory
agencies. At EPA, the risk assessment units in the
Office of Health and Environmental Assessment of the
Office of Research and Development prepare assessments
for regulatory program offices that are organizationally
under different assistant administrators. However, the
Office of Toxic Substances does its own assessments, and
several other program offices are responsible for their
own exposure assessments. The risk assessments for the
FDA'S Bureau of Foods are produced within the Bureau, but
by an office distinct from offices responsible for formulating regulations and enforcement; since 1976, the Directorate of Health Standards Programs in OSHA has both
performed risk assessments and formulated all early risk
management options. Different agencies also have success-

fully used different organizational arrangements for risk
assessment. FDA, for example, has often called on NRC
and NTP for assessments, but in other cases relied on its
own staff. The Committee's review of different agency
structures and procedures did not demonstrate that one
particular structure produced risk assessments of superior
quality and integrity. In addition, the Committee notes
that, even if there were a clear finding that a particular
arrangement works for a given agency or program, it would
be extremely difficult (given the diversity in agency and
program mandates, personnel needs, and histories) to
justify a suggestion that that arrangement would best
serve all agencies or programs.

2. <u>Organizational separation has several important
   drawbacks that are likely to be intensified with
   increasing degrees of separation.</u>

There are several arguments against organizational
separation. Separation of the risk assessment function
from an agency's regulatory activities is likely to
inhibit the interaction between assessors and regulators
that is necessary for the proper interpretation of risk
estimates and the evaluation of risk management options.
Separation can lead to disjunction between assessment and
regulatory agendas and cause delays in regulatory proceedings. Common sense suggests that increased separation
would aggravate these drawbacks. In its review, the Committee observed these disadvantages when assessors and
regulators were in different organizations (e.g., NIOSH
and NRC). Another perceived drawback in extra-agency
separation that was neither detected nor likely to emerge
in the Committee's review is the erosion of scientific
competence within agency staffs if risk assessments are
routinely performed outside the agency. Also, any major
organizational change may have a disruptive effect on
agency performance; thus, such organizational changes are
especially questionable when the benefits, if any, are
unclear.

3. <u>Organizational arrangements that separate risk
   assessment from risk management decision-making will
   not necessarily ensure that the policy basis of
   choices made in the risk assessment process is clearly
   distinguished from the scientific basis of such
   choices.</u>

If risk assessment as practiced by the regulatory
agencies were pure science, perhaps an organizational
separation could effectively sharpen the distinction
between science and policy in risk assessment and regulatory decision-making. However, many of the analytic
choices made throughout the risk assessment process
require individual judgments that are based on both scientific and policy considerations. The policy considerations in risk assessment are of a different character
from those involved in specific risk management decisions
and are generally common to all assessments for similar
health effects. Thus, even when one has drawn the relatively obvious distinction between risk assessment and
risk management, there remains the more difficult task of
distinguishing between the science and policy dimensions
of risk assessment itself. We believe that the latter
distinction cannot be ensured or maintained through organizational arrangements. Given the inherent mixture of
science and policy in risk assessment, organizational
separation would simply move risk assessment policy into
a different organization that would then have to become
politically accountable. The Committee believes that
other approaches are more likely to maintain the distinction between science and policy in risk assessment, most
notably the development of and adherence to guidelines.

VALUE OF CENTRALIZATION

4. Common risk assessments performed primarily by scientists from all interested agencies on an ad hoc basis
   may capture the major advantages of centralization
   without the drawbacks that accompany permanent,
   extra-agency centralization.

An argument often advanced for centralization is that
it might expedite and perhaps reduce the administrative
costs of decision-making when two or more agencies contemplate regulation of the same substance. And if two or
more agencies are going to regulate the same substance,
there is much to be said for developing a system that
facilitates production of a single, common risk assessment. This was one rationale for CPSC's decision to
empanel a group of scientists to evaluate the carcinogenicity data on formaldehyde, and it argues in support of
the central panels suggested in H.R. 638 and the American
Industrial Health Council's proposal. Although the Com-

mittee endorses government-wide consistency in risk
assessment, it is less sanguine concerning the prospects
of a permanent arrangement for such centralized risk
assessment as contemplated by these proposals, in which
the idea of centralized assessment is inextricably linked
to extra-agency separation. The Committee concluded that
extra-agency separation would have disadvantages that
would offset any advantages.

The Committee did find, however, that agency scientists
could collaborate to perform joint risk assessments on an
ad hoc basis. Because agency scientists would perform an
assessment, such an arrangement would avoid most of the
drawbacks of extra-agency separation. The Committee
looked at the Panel on Formaldehyde as an example of a
centralized assessment group. In the Committee's view,
the Panel functioned well and produced an assessment that
has been accepted by the scientific community. The
Panel's assessment has not produced parallel regulatory
action among the agencies, and the Committee observed
that similar risk assessments should not necessarily lead
to similar regulatory decisions, which reflect considerations that often justify different risk management
responses.

USE OF SCIENTIFIC REVIEW PANELS

5. Independent scientific review of agency risk
   assessments improves the scientific quality of the
   assessments and strengthens them against later
   challenge.

Agencies and programs with mandated peer review panels,
such as EPA's Office of Pesticide Programs, which is
required to submit to a Scientific Advisory Panel proposals to cancel or restrict pesticide use, produce final
risk assessments in support of regulatory decisions that
are generally of high scientific quality and are accepted
by the public and the regulated parties. In contrast,
the Committee found several cases in which mechanisms for
peer review could be markedly improved: OSHA, which uses
public comments to refine its risk assessments, rather
than formal peer review; NIOSH, which has not had a mechanism to ensure that reviewers' comments are given appropriate consideration; and FDA's Bureau of Foods, which
uses ad hoc panels to review its assessments (a procedure
that unfortunately can be circumvented).

• <u>Standing and continuing review panels that have</u>
<u>mechanisms to maintain the independence of their</u>
<u>members appear to be the most useful review bodies.</u>
Continuity and independence of review panels help to
ensure that such panels are sensitive to regulatory needs
while retaining the necessary scientific objectivity.
Examples of standing committees, such as the Scientific
Advisory Panel in EPA, support this perception. Conversely, the Committee observed that short-lived or ad
hoc groups, such as the Subcommittee on Airborne Carcinogens, often do not have sufficient time to develop a
working relationship among panel members and that much of
the time allotted to review is actually spent in clarify-
ing individual versus panel viewpoints and understandings.
Similarly, an ad hoc panel may not clearly understand its
role in relation to the regulatory process. Thus, standing panels appear to be of greater value to the agency
than ad hoc committees. Furthermore, the existence of a
standing panel might encourage an agency to seek its
advice more frequently.

Because it is important for review committees to be
free to express their scientific judgments without
concern for regulatory implications, panels that are
formed in a manner that neither compromises nor appears
to compromise their independence are more likely to
improve ultimate risk assessments. The Committee observed
that several review panels used by EPA already have a
nomination process that places the responsibility for
developing a slate of possible panel members outside the
agency. Although the EPA Administrator makes the final
selections of panel members, the fact that nominations
come from outside the agency emphasizes the intent that
EPA panels be independent and as free of agency influence
as possible. A related point is that membership on EPA
panels, and in fact on most review panels used by the
regulatory agencies, rotates; members are usually selected
for staggered, fixed terms (generally 3-4 years). This
rotation itself reduces the likelihood that members will
develop an institutional bias.

• <u>Review panels are best qualified to give scien-</u>
<u>tific advice when they are composed of scientists who</u>
<u>are highly knowledgeable in the appropriate</u>
<u>disciplines.</u>
For carcinogenicity risk assessments, for example,
some relevant disciplines would be toxicology, pathology,
biostatistics, chemistry, and epidemiology. The Com-

mittee believes that professional or organizational affiliation should not be used as a primary criterion in the determination of the makeup of a particular panel. That is, in contrast with the advisory panels used by OSHA, which are constituted to reflect balance among different affiliations and presumed biases, the Committee believes that scientific competence must be the primary factor determining panel membership if review panels are to be asked to give their advice on the scientific aspects of an agency's risk assessments. However, the Committee notes that panel members who understand the policy implications of their scientific judgments are more likely to be helpful to an agency's assessment process and that an attempt to balance viewpoints of scientifically qualified panel members may increase a panel's credibility.

* Review panels will be most effective if they have the authority to review agency risk assessments before announcement of the agency's intended regulatory actions, except in cases of emergency.

The Committee believes that review panels serving regulatory agencies should serve in an advisory capacity. That is, the judgments of a panel should not be binding on the agency. Nevertheless, the Committee also believes that the authority of agency review panels should be such that agencies must demonstrate that adequate consideration has been given to reviewers' judgments, and prior consultation with review panels helps to ensure this. Because announcements of intended actions or proposed regulations must be thoroughly developed and substantiated, review at the time of announcement or later is likely to be too late to influence an agency; although the regulation is only proposed, the decision of whether to act has, for all practical purposes, already been made. In the Committee's judgment, exceptions to this idea of prior review are appropriate in the case of emergency actions, such as suspension of pesticide registration. Risk assessments supporting such actions could be reviewed after the announced action.

* Independent panels with authority to review risk assessments for all agency regulatory decisions, including decisions not to act, are more likely to ensure that agency decisions rest on valid scientific grounds.

Panels with the authority to request the review of any agency risk assessment supporting a particular regulatory decision will have a greater impact on agency decision-making. For example, if a panel can review only assessments referred to it by an agency, some agency decisions might not benefit from independent review of their scientific basis. This is especially likely if an agency has decided not to regulate. Such a decision may have considerable impact and should receive the same careful review as decisions to regulate. In addition, panels with the authority to request reviews can respond to suggestions for review from the public.

* **Although most requirements of the Federal Advisory Committee Act are salutary, others may inhibit agency use of review panels.**

The Committee believes that most provisions of the Act are beneficial and endorses such provisions as the requirement that advisory committees meet in public and provide advance notice of their meetings. However, the Act does impose requirements, some burdensome, for agency-created bodies that meet the definition of advisory committee. Notably, the Act requires that an advisory committee be formally chartered by an agency head and approved by the General Services Administration. This procedure has often proved cumbersome. Some agencies, such as FDA, lack independent chartering authority and thus require approval at the departmental level. In addition, procedures used by the General Services Administration for screening new committees have often imposed long delays, sometimes inspired by political concerns about committee membership or by resistance to the creation of new government "agencies." These legal requirements of the Act have caused some agencies to seek other ways of obtaining the views of scientific experts, especially when the issues involve single chemicals or tests. In such cases, regulators often confine their consultations to government scientists, who can be accessible immediately and, if necessary, for extended periods.

* **Written reviews help to ensure agency consideration of scientific criticism.**

A summary of a panel's review that is transmitted in written form and made available to the public will help to avoid confusion and to ensure agency consideration of the panel's comments. As mentioned earlier, in the absence of adequate mechanisms to ensure agency consideration of reviewers' comments, the comments might be ignored, or the public might perceive that they are ignored. Putting its summary in writing should also ensure that the panel states its findings clearly and make it more likely that the agency will interpret its comments correctly.

OTHER OBSERVATIONS

6. Preparation of fully documented written risk assessments that explicitly define the judgments made and attendant uncertainties clarifies the agency decision-making process and aids the review process considerably.

When a fully documented written risk assessment is not produced before an agency's decision to regulate or not to regulate, it is difficult to understand the process by which an agency made its assessment. The Committee believes that the creation of such a document encourages public understanding of and respect for agency procedures and provides a basis for review by a scientific advisory panel. Furthermore, a detailed risk assessment document that clearly identifies the inference options chosen in the assessment and explains the rationale for those choices will help to maintain a sharper distinction between science and policy in the assessment of risk and will guard against the inappropriate intrusion of risk management considerations.

REFERENCES

AIHC (American Industrial Health Council). 1979. Recommended Framework for Identifying Carcinogens and Regulating Them in Manufacturing Situations.
EPA (Environmental Protection Agency). 1976. Health risk and economic impact assessments of suspected carcinogens: interim procedures and guidelines. Fed. Reg. 41(102):21402-21405.
EPA (Environmental Protection Agency). 1979. Water Quality Criteria, Request for Comments. Fed. Reg. 44(52):15926.
EPA (Environmental Protection Agency). 1980. Water Quality Criteria Documents; Availability. Fed. Reg. 45(231):79350-79353.

Food Safety Council. Social and Economic Committee. 1979. Principles and Processes for Making Food Safety Decisions. 54 pp.

Higginson, John. 1982. Report of the Scientific Workshop on the Critical Evaluation of Proposals by the American Industrial Health Council to Strengthen the Scientific Base for Regulatory Decisions.

Kantrowitz, Arthur. 1975. Controlling technology democratically. Am. Sci. 63:505-509.

NRC (National Research Council). 1981. The Handling of Risk Assessments in NRC Reports. A Report to the Governing Board, National Research Council, by the Governing Board Committee on the Assessment of Risk. 19 pp.

Office of Science and Technology Policy. 1978. Identification, Characterization, and Control of Potential Human Carcinogens: A Framework for Federal Decision-Making.

U.S. Congress. 1981a. Omnibus Budget Reconciliation Act. (P.L. 97-35, August 13, 1981) 15 U.S.C. 2077.

U.S. Congress. 1981b. House of Representatives, Committee on Agriculture, Hearings on the National Science Council Act, H.R. 638. Hearings Before the Subcommittee on Department Operations, Research, and Foreign Agriculture of the Committee on Agriculture, June 23, 1981.

U.S. Congress. 1981c. House of Representatives H.R. 638. National Science Council Act 97th Congress, 1st Session, 1981.

U.S. Congress. 1981d. Senate. S. 1442. Food Safety Amendments of 1981, 97th Congress, 1st Session, 1981.

IV
Recommendations

The Committee has reviewed federal risk assessment for hazards to public health, particularly for chemically induced cancer, and has presented its findings concerning the nature of risk assessment, the nature and utility of risk inference guidelines, and the effects of alternative organizational arrangements on risk assessment. The Committee's review leads to the general observation that the process of risk assessment, as performed by and for federal regulatory agencies, has been developing rapidly in recent years, both with respect to its scientific basis and with respect to the agencies' organizational arrangements. Change this rapid is bound to lead to misunderstanding about the use of risk assessment in regulatory policy-making, particularly if some misconstrue risk assessment to be a strictly scientific undertaking. Much of the criticism of risk assessment stems from dissatisfaction with regulatory outcomes, and many proposals for change are based largely on the unwarranted assumption that altering the administrative arrangements for risk assessment would lead to regulatory outcomes that critics will find less disagreeable. Because risk assessment is only one aspect of risk management decision-making, however, even greatly improved assessments will not eliminate dissatisfaction with risk management decisions.

The Committee believes that the basic problem with risk assessment is not its administrative setting, but rather the sparseness and uncertainty of the scientific knowledge of the health hazards addressed. Reorganization of the risk assessment function will not create the data and underlying knowledge that assessors need to make risk assessments more precise. We hold that the most productive path to a solution has three parts:

* Implementation of procedural changes that ensure that risk assessments take full advantage of the available scientific knowledge while maintaining the diverse organizational approaches to administration of risk assessment needed to accommodate the varied requirements of federal regulatory programs.
* Standardization of analytic procedures among federal programs through the development and use of uniform inference guidelines.
* Creation of a mechanism that will ensure orderly, continuing review and modification of risk assessment procedures as scientific understanding of hazards improves.

The Committee offers in the following pages 10 recommendations whose implementation it believes will meet these general objectives.

IMPROVING RISK ASSESSMENT THROUGH PROCEDURAL CHANGES

RECOMMENDATION 1

Regulatory agencies should take steps to establish and maintain a clear conceptual distinction between assessment of risks and the consideration of risk management alternatives; that is, the scientific findings and policy judgments embodied in risk assessments should be explicitly distinguished from the political, economic, and technical considerations that influence the design and choice of regulatory strategies.

Although the Committee concludes that risk assessment cannot be made completely free of policy considerations, it also believes that policy associated with specific risk management decisions should not influence risk assessment unduly. Risk assessment and risk management involve different goals, kinds of expertness, and operating principles. The goal of risk assessment is to describe, as accurately as possible, the possible health consequences of changes in human exposure to a hazardous substance; the need for accuracy implies that the best available scientific knowledge, supplemented as necessary by assumptions that are consistent with science, will be applied. The ultimate aim of risk management is to evaluate trade-offs between health consequences and other effects of specific regulatory actions; this evaluation includes the application of value judgments to reach a policy decision.

Experience shows the difficulties that can arise from
a blurring of the distinction between the two elements.
If risk management considerations (for example, the economic or political effects of a particular control action
for a particular chemical) are seen to affect either the
scientific interpretations or the choice of inference
options in a risk assessment, the credibility of the
assessment inside and outside the agency can be compro-
mised, and the risk management decision itself may lose
legitimacy. Indeed, such consequences can flow from the
mere perception, as well as the fact, of such influences.
Each regulatory agency should commit itself to safeguarding the distinction between the processes of risk assessment and risk management. One among several suggestions
for accomplishing this safeguarding is to restructure the
formal organization, separating an agency's or program's
risk assessment staff from its policy-making staff, possibly by establishing a separate risk assessment unit
outside the agency. The Committee does not, however,
recommend that agencies use any particular organizational
arrangement for risk assessment. One might surmise that
separating the staffs would help to reduce the likelihood
that risk management considerations will influence risk
assessment, but our survey of agency structures provided
no clear evidence that such an influence was related to
the degree of administrative separation.

Formal separation has disadvantages that must be balanced against its value in maintaining a distinction
between risk assessment and risk management. Risk assessment and risk management functions are analytically distinct, but in practice they do--and must--interact.
Organizational arrangements that completely isolate risk
assessors from regulatory policy-makers may inhibit important communication in both directions. For example, to
complete risk characterization, risk assessors must know
what policy options are to be used to calculate alternative projected exposures, and new options may develop as
the risk management process proceeds. Moreover, direct
communication with the risk assessors is desirable to
ensure that the regulatory decision-maker understands the
relative quality of the available scientific evidence,
the degree of uncertainty implicit in the final risk
assessment, and the sensitivity of the results to the
assumptions that have been necessary to produce the
assessment. Such separation could also impair the risk
manager's ability to obtain assessments that are timely
and in a useful form. The advisability of organizational

separation hinges on comparison of its benefits and costs in particular agencies and programs.

Because drawbacks are likely to be most pronounced in the case of extra-agency separation, the Committee does not believe that it is appropriate to remove the risk assessment function and place it in an organization completely separated from the regulatory agencies, as is contemplated in the AIHC proposal and H.R. 638. This judgment is supported by the conclusion that the benefits of increased separation are uncertain and that the disruption and confusion caused by reorganization could be considerable.

Measures other than organizational separation can ensure the distinction between the assessment of risk and the consideration of risk management alternatives. These measures include the practice of preparing written risk assessments (Recommendation 2), arranging for independent peer review (Recommendation 3), and adhering to uniform guidelines for risk assessment (Recommendations 5 through 9).

RECOMMENDATION 2

Before an agency decides whether a substance should or should not be regulated as a health hazard, a detailed and comprehensive written risk assessment should be prepared and made publicly accessible. This written assessment should clearly distinguish between the scientific basis and the policy basis for the agency's conclusions.

Although agencies commonly perform risk assessments before they take regulatory actions, the written assessments that are prepared vary in coverage, amount of explanatory detail, format, and completeness to an extent that limits their use as instruments of communication. The Committee believes that the matters addressed are so important and the consequences so far-reaching that a written risk assessment should be prepared for every significant regulatory decision and that each should be a clear, detailed, and comprehensive account of the analysis performed. A written assessment should describe the volume and weight of scientific evidence to help to clarify the scientific and policy bases for regulatory decisions.

The written assessment should be made accessible to the public at a time and in a form that facilitates public participation in any attendant risk management decision.

The Committee believes that the requirement to prepare a written assessment imposes a salutary discipline that, for several reasons, will improve the performance of risk assessment. First, the requirement to prepare a comprehensive written assessment will encourage the agency to explain how each component of the assessment was treated; that should minimize the likelihood that risk management considerations will, unnoticed, affect the outcome of the assessment. Second, a written assessment can help to distinguish the factual basis of a risk assessment from inferences drawn where there is a lack of scientific consensus; this distinction will facilitate scientific review of the risk assessment, document the scientific basis of the assessment for outside observers, and acquaint the regulatory decision-maker with the relative completeness of the scientific evidence. Third, it will aid communication among specialists working on different parts of the assessment. Fourth, the existence of an explicit description should simplify the conduct of later assessments of the same chemical, if additional scientific evidence comes to light or other regulatory programs review the same substance. Finally, written risk assessments will be useful to institutions that oversee regulatory agencies, notably Congress and those responsible for judicial review. It is important, however, that the format and scope of written assessments not become an independent basis for legal attack.

Content and Form

An agency's written risk assessment should set forth in detail the nature and quality of the relevant scientific evidence concerning the substance in question and should cover all relevant components of risk assessment. It should reflect attention to any applicable guidelines relied on in interpreting the evidence, so that a reader can ascertain what inference options were used, and should describe the scientific rationale for any departures from methods prescribed in such guidelines. If the choice of inference options is not governed by guidelines, the written assessment itself should make explicit the assumptions used to interpret data or support conclusions reached in the absence of data. The document should acknowledge gaps and uncertainties in available information.

An agency's written assessments are likely to prove most useful if they follow a consistent format, so that readers, once familiar with the format, can use them efficiently. We believe that each program or agency can establish a uniform structure for its written assessments, and we hope that similarity, if not uniformity, will be possible in written assessments prepared throughout the government.

Actions Covered

This recommendation is not intended to apply to the risk posed by every substance, use, or exposure that engages an agency's attention. It is intended to apply to agency decisions concerning important human exposure to a hazard. Such decisions would include (but not be limited to) establishment of an occupational safety and health standard by OSHA, cancellation by EPA of the federal registration of a pesticide to which there is widespread human exposure, and EPA promulgation of limits for an air or water pollutant. The categories of actions covered by this recommendation could be defined precisely only after detailed statutory analysis. EPA appears to have had satisfactory experience with the practice of classifying its regulations as "major" (those with very large economic and other effects that require an extensive regulatory analysis and formal review by the Office of Management and Budget), "significant" (a larger category defined by internal EPA criteria), and "minor" (a similarly large group of routine and technical actions). We suggest that EPA prepare a written assessment for every major and significant action, and we encourage other agencies to devise similar methods of identifying which regulatory actions require written assessments.

An agency's decision to refrain from regulation can often have important consequences, both for health and for the economy, and such decisions should rest on accurate, objective assessments of risk. The denial of a petition to act on a chemical to which exposure is extensive is an example. When an agency is confronted with choosing between limiting exposures to a substance and taking some lesser action and there is serious dispute over the character or extent of the risk posed, a written assessment is advisable.

RECOMMENDATION 3

An agency's risk assessment should be reviewed by an
independent science advisory panel before any major
regulatory action or decision not to regulate. Peer
review may be performed by science panels already
established or authorized under current law or, in their
absence, by panels created for this purpose.

    • If an agency's workload is substantial, a
standing advisory panel (or panels) should be established
to review its risk assessments; otherwise, ad hoc panels
should be established on a case-by-case basis.
    • Panel members should be selected for their
scientific or technical competence.
    • The appointment of members should be the
responsibility of each agency director, but nominations
from the public and scientific organizations should be
invited, unless current law prescribes another procedure.
    • Panels should provide to the referring agencies
written evaluations of agency risk assessments, and the
evaluations should be available for public inspection.

    This recommendation endorses outside peer review of
agency risk assessments. Such review should contribute
to the important distinction between risk assessment and
risk management, because risk management information
would be excluded from the review; should improve the
scientific quality of the assessments through the process
of criticism and response; and should increase the credibility of agency assessments. The practice of preparing
written risk assessments will facilitate the review
process.
    The peer review function that we visualize is already
evident in some agencies. We believe that a single
approach would not fit all contexts, but that any mechanism for scientific peer review should meet the general
criteria described below.

Panel Form

The review function we recommend could be performed
effectively by an appropriately qualified standing panel
of independent scientists that is responsible for reviewing agency assessments of a particular class of hazards.
Any agency program responsible for a large number of

157

compounds to which humans are exposed in large amounts seems to be an appropriate candidate for a standing scientific review panel, but some programs may deal with so few chronic health hazards that a standing panel is not warranted. The Committee specifically contemplates that the review function recommended here can be performed by panels already available to several agency programs.

Panel Composition and Selection

Members of a scientific review panel should be selected for their competence in fields relevant to the assessment of risks of the kind being evaluated. In our judgment, employees of private business organizations, members of environmental groups, and government research or regulatory agency employees should not necessarily be disqualified; but no panel members should be employees of the agency whose risk assessments are to be reviewed, nor should any members participate in the review of substances in which they or their employers have substantial economic or other interests or on whose risks they or their employers have publicly taken a position. It is important to safeguard both the reality and the appearance of complete objectivity for each review.

We contemplate that, as is common for existing panels, the appointing official would be the head of the agency whose risk assessments are to be reviewed. Such an arrangement could be thought to jeopardize a panel's independence from the agency, particularly in cases in which it is known which chemicals the panel will review. Accordingly, each agency should establish procedures for obtaining nominees for panel membership whose objectivity is ensured. For example, some current procedures call for agency selection of members from lists of nominees provided by the President of the National Academy of Sciences and by the Directors of the National Institutes of Health and the National Science Foundation. We see no magic in any particular nomination process. The important objective is a process that, first, ensures that panel members are selected for their training and experience in relevant fields; second, prevents the appointing official from forming a panel that will produce (or appear to produce) a predetermined result; and, third, operates expeditiously. We recommend that this process include an opportunity for members of the public to nominate persons for panel membership.

Panel Functions

Our recommendation contemplates that, in a typical case,
the responsible agency will have prepared a written
assessment of the risk posed by a substance. The independent scientific panel would be asked to review that
assessment for comprehensiveness, scientific accuracy,
and consistency with any applicable risk assessment
guidelines. If such guidelines are flexible, an important panel function will be to ensure that departures
from the inference options favored by the guidelines are
justified on scientific grounds. In performing this role,
the panel should, if it desires, have access to all the
data available to the agency, including those on which
the agency's analysts relied, as well as the agency's
written assessment. The panel should subject the agency's
risk assessment to such scrutiny as the members find
necessary to satisfy themselves that it is, with or without revisions, as complete and objective as available
data permit. The panel should provide a written evaluation of the agency's risk assessment, including recommendations for revision, if appropriate. This evaluation
should be available for public examination by the time
the agency initiates public proceedings to alter human
exposure to the substance in question for example, when
the agency issues a notice of proposed rule-making.

Panel Agenda

Independent review of agency risk assessments is designed
to ensure the integrity and quality of the scientific
bases for regulatory decisions affecting human health.
Therefore, the Committee recommends that every action,
including a decision not to regulate, that requires a
written risk assessment be available for independent
scientific review. A scientific review panel's agenda
may also include risk assessments for other decisions of
interest to panel members, or its review could be
initiated after a request by a third party. In the
latter case, panels should have the authority to decide
whether or not to respond to such requests for review.
In general, the Committee expects that the panels would
exercise discretion in invoking their authority to review
assessments for routine, minor actions.

Timing of Review

Independent scientific review of agency risk assessments
should occur before an agency commences the public process
leading to regulatory action. The purpose is to expose
the agency's initial assessment of the risk posed by a
substance to expert scrutiny at a time when review can
influence the agency's course of action. Experience
suggests that agencies are less receptive to criticism of
the basis of their actions after they have announced a
proposed course of action. Furthermore, although independent review can sometimes forestall misguided regulatory actions even after they are initiated, prior review
of such actions may help to avoid serious damage to agency
credibility and unnecessary costs to private interests
that would be adversely affected by public proposals for
regulatory action. We recognize an important exception
to our general recommendation of preaction peer review.
Several statutes expressly empower agencies to act in an
emergency to curtail human exposure to a substance that
poses a serious health risk. Agencies have also devised
informal procedures to effect immediate protection of
humans exposed to dangerous substances in other contexts.
Our recommendation is not intended to cast doubt on the
legitimacy of such authority or to impede its appropriate
exercise. When an agency concludes that a hazard warrants
immediate regulatory action to limit human exposure, it
should be able to take action consistent with existing
law without first going through the review process that
we recommend. Promptly thereafter, however, the agency
should submit its written risk assessment for independent
review in accordance with the procedures outlined here.

Weight of Panel Evaluation

A scientific review panel's critique of an agency's risk
assessment should not be binding; that is, the agency
should not be obliged to revise its risk assessment if
the panel regards it as deficient. Agencies have a
responsibility to state the basis of their actions, and
the authority for their actions must remain their own.
Serious panel criticism, however, would in practice cause
any agency at least to reconsider, and ordinarily to
revise, its risk assessment. The agency should discuss
any important criticisms of its assessment in its proposed
regulatory action, and its response to a panel's criti-

cisms would be an appropriate subject for public comment, as well as a possible basis for judicial challenge to any final action.

We believe that an important benefit of peer review occurs before the review begins: risk assessors who expect an assessment to be subjected to serious scrutiny by eminent qualified reviewers are likely to be more careful and clear about the use and limits of scientific evidence.

Federal Advisory Committee Act

The Federal Advisory Committee Act imposes many salutary requirements on panels established to advise federal agencies, including notably the requirement that panel meetings be held in public. But the Act's requirement that new advisory committees be chartered by the General Services Administration imposes substantial delays and its requirement that panel meetings be announced in the Federal Register at least 15 days in advance can markedly slow a panel's work. Consideration should be given to modifying both requirements or exempting such panels from the Act, as Congress did for CPSC's Chronic Hazard Advisory Panels.

RECOMMENDATION 4

When two or more agencies share interest in and jurisdiction over a health hazard that is a candidate for regulation by them in the near term, a joint risk assessment should be prepared under the auspices of the National Toxicology Program or another appropriate organization. Joint risk assessments should be prepared primarily by scientific personnel provided by the agencies and assisted as necessary by other government scientists.

This recommendation endorses coordination in assessing the risks of chemicals that are likely candidates for regulation by two or more agencies. Although all the end uses of a substance may fall within the jurisdiction of one agency (such as FDA for a food additive), exposures occurring during production, transportation, and distribution usually are within other agencies' jurisdictions. Thus, chemicals that pose a hazard to human health are at least theoretically subject to regulation by two or more federal agencies. The Committee agrees with proponents of the centralization of risk assessment responsibilities that the agencies involved should operate on the basis of a common assessment of the substance's risks. However, the Committee differs with respect to the method for achieving this end.

Actions Covered

Our recommendation does not call for the performance of a joint risk assessment in every instance in which a substance potentially falls within the jurisdiction of two or more agencies; we limit our proposal to circumstances in which assessment by more than one agency is likely in the near future. This limitation has two rationales. First, substantial risk may be associated with routes of exposure of concern to only one agency. Under such circumstances, it would be unreasonable to invest time and resources to establish an interagency panel of scientists. Second, even if different types of exposure entail risks, a substance may legitimately rank low in priority for one agency and high for another.

Placement and Procedures

The approach we visualize is similar to that followed in 1980, when the Interagency Regulatory Liaison Group, at the suggestion of CPSC, sought the assistance of the National Toxicology Program to examine the carcinogenicity of formaldehyde. The Program formed an ad hoc panel that consisted entirely of government scientists, including some from EPA, OSHA, and FDA.

We suggest that the National Toxicology Program be the usual vehicle for coordinating preparation of joint risk assessments. The National Toxicology Program has been in operation for several years and, in the Committee's judgment, has performed capably as coordinator of federal toxicologic research. It has displayed an ability to command the service of the government's best scientists. And it has developed effective working relationships with the regulatory agencies, which have become accustomed to looking to it for assistance in evaluating substances that are candidates for regulation.

We expect that suggestions for establishment of an interagency task force to evaluate a hazard will come

from the interested regulatory agencies. The personnel
assigned to assemble the relevant data and perform the
assessment could include scientists from the interested
regulatory agencies, including the initiating agencies,
and scientists from government research organizations,
such as the National Institute of Environmental Health
Sciences, the National Cancer Institute, and the National
Center for Toxicological Research. The Committee recommends that task forces follow the same guidelines used by
the regulatory agencies. Joint risk assessments should
be subjected to independent scientific review.

For reasons presented in the discussion of Recommendation 1, the Committee believes that such an ad hoc
approach is preferable to creation of a centralized risk
assessment body.

IMPROVING RISK ASSESSMENT THROUGH UNIFORM INFERENCE GUIDELINES

RECOMMENDATION 5

Uniform inference guidelines should be developed for the
use of federal regulatory agencies in the risk assessment
process.

In the Committee's judgment, the development of uniform
inference guidelines is feasible and desirable. However,
the Committee emphasizes that guidelines cannot provide a
formula for automatically calculating risk from available
data; case-by-case scientific interpretation will still
be crucial, and risk assessments must reflect experts'
characterizations of the quality of the data and of the
uncertainty associated with the final assessment.

Adherence to uniform guidelines has several advantages
over ad hoc performance of risk assessments. Guidelines
could help to separate risk assessment from risk management considerations, improve public understanding of the
process, foster consistency, and prevent oversights and
judgments that are inconsistent with current scientific
thought. The development and application of guidelines
would help to focus discussion by the public and the
scientific community on the generic issues of risk
assessment, outside the sometimes charged context of
particular regulatory decisions. Such discussion could
stimulate research interest and lead to evolutionary
improvement in the guidelines and thus in the quality of

risk assessment--improvement that would not occur if risk
assessments were performed on an ad hoc basis. Guidelines
also provide an efficient means to ensure the quality and
relevance of data generated in new bioassay, epidemiologic, and other pertinent studies on the toxicity of
particular chemicals, thus improving the scientific data
base for future risk assessments of those chemicals.
Guidelines can also help regulated parties to know in
advance the criteria that agencies will apply in evaluating substances. Industry would benefit if all federal
agencies used the same guidelines. Furthermore, uniform
federal guidelines could help to harmonize the current
development of risk assessment methods by an increasing
number of state programs.

Uniform guidelines should be prepared for hazard
identification, dose-response assessment, and risk characterization. Government-wide guidelines for exposure
assessment may be impractical, and this aspect of risk
assessment is treated separately in Recommendation 9.

The Committee is aware of several arguments to the
effect that uniform guidelines could have adverse effects.
We believe, however, that well-designed and carefully
applied guidelines will minimize these disadvantages.

RECOMMENDATION 6

The inference guidelines should be comprehensive,
detailed, and flexible. They should make explicit the
distinctions between the science and policy aspects of
risk assessment. Specifically, they should have the
following characteristics:

•   They should describe all components of hazard
identification, dose-response assessment, and risk
characterization and should require assessors to show
that they have considered all the necessary components in
each step.
•   They should provide detailed guidance on how each
component should be considered, but permit flexibility to
depart from the general case if an assessor demonstrates
that an exception is warranted on scientific grounds.
•   They should provide specific guidance on
components of data evaluation that require the imposition
of risk assessment policy decisions and should clearly
distinguish those decisions from scientific decisions.

• They should provide specific guidance on how an
assessor is to present the results of the assessment and
the attendant uncertainties.

Distinguishing Science from Policy

A frequent deficiency of agency risk assessments is the
failure to distinguish between scientific and policy
considerations in risk assessment. Critics contend that
the results of risk assessment are often seen as scientific findings by regulators and the public, whereas in
fact they are based in part on other considerations. The
Committee believes that guidelines can lead to risk
assessments that clearly delineate the limits of current
scientific knowledge and the policy basis for choosing
among inference options.

Comprehensive and Detailed Nature

Comprehensive, detailed guidelines are needed to delineate
risk assessment as a process distinct from risk management. Comprehensive guidelines are those which address
all components of risk assessment that are subject to
generic treatment. Detailed guidelines are those which
provide substantial supplementary scientific discussion
of each component. Such discussion helps to reduce the
possibility that analysts will misuse guidelines as
cookbook instructions and helps analysts to anticipate
special conditions for which particular inference options
are appropriate or inappropriate.

Broad statements of principle are inadequate, because
they leave components undefined and may permit excessive
discretion in particular cases. An explicit, comprehensive statement has the advantages of improving public
understanding of government risk assessment and of
assisting regulated parties to anticipate government
actions.

Another reason for specifying comprehensive, detailed
guidelines is that they hold the greatest promise of
preventing inconsistency within and among agencies. At
numerous points in a risk assessment, different risk
assessors may select different (but scientifically valid)
inference options; guidelines should specifically address
each of these. A related advantage is an improvement in
quality control that could occur if all assessors were

required to consider the broad range of issues addressed in such guidelines; that would decrease the likelihood that important considerations would be neglected or that uninformed judgment would occur.

Flexibility

The Committee espouses flexible guidelines. Rigid guidelines, which permit no variation, might preclude the consideration of relevant scientific information peculiar to a particular chemical and thus force assessors to use inference options that are not appropriate in a given case. Also, rigid guidelines might mandate the continued use of concepts that become obsolete with new scientific developments. Large segments of the scientific community would undoubtedly object to such guidelines as incompatible with the use of the best scientific judgment for policy decisions.

Flexibility can be introduced by the incorporation of default options. The assessor would be instructed to use a designated (default) option unless specific scientific evidence suggested otherwise. The guidelines would thus permit exceptions to the general case, as long as each exception could be justified scientifically. Such justifications would be reviewed by the scientific review panels and by the public under procedures described above. Guidelines could profitably highlight subjects undergoing relatively rapid scientific development (e.g., the use of metabolic data for interspecies comparisons) and any other components in which exceptions to particular default options were likely to arise. They should also attempt to present criteria for evaluating whether an exception is justified.

Presenting the Results of the Assessment

Conclusions based on a large number of sequential, discretionary choices necessarily entail a large, cumulative uncertainty. The degree of uncertainty may be masked to some extent when, in the final form of an assessment, risk is presented as a number with an associated measure of statistical significance. If they are to be most instructive to decision-makers, assessments should provide some insight into qualitative characteristics of the data and interpretations that may impute more or less certainty to the final results.

RECOMMENDATION 7

The process for developing, adopting, applying, and revising the recommended inference guidelines for risk assessment should reflect their dual scientific and policy nature:

• An expert board should be established to develop recommended guidelines for consideration and adoption by regulatory agencies. The board's recommended guidelines should define the scientific capabilities and limitations in assessing health risks, delineate subjects of uncertainty, and define the consequences of alternative policies for addressing the uncertainties.
• The expert board's report and recommendations should be submitted to the agencies responsible for regulating the hazards addressed by the guidelines for their evaluation and adoption. The agencies, perhaps with central coordination, should, when possible, choose a preferred option from among the options that are consistent with current scientific understanding. The procedures for adoption should afford an opportunity for members of the public to comment.
• The process followed by the government for adoption of inference guidelines should ensure that the resulting guidelines are uniform among all responsible agencies and are consistently adhered to in assessing the risks of individual hazards.
• The resulting uniform guidelines should govern the performance of risk assessments by all the agencies that adopt them until they are re-examined and revised; they should not prevent members of the public from disputing their soundness or applicability in particular cases. In short, the guidelines should have the status of established agency procedures, rather than binding regulations.
• The guidelines should be reviewed periodically with the advice and recommendations of the expert board. The process for revising the guidelines, like the process for adoption, should afford an opportunity for comment by all interested individuals and organizations.

Inference guidelines for risk assessment are based largely on science, but other considerations are involved in components with substantial scientific uncertainty. For these, the choice among inference options can have substantial policy ramifications. Thus, we recommend a two-step process in which a board of experts recommends guidelines and provides scientific commentary on available inference options and then the government adopts final guidelines based in part on the board's recommendations.

The Board and Its Role

The recommended guidelines should be developed by a congressionally chartered board of experts who are independent of regulatory policy-making. We describe this board, its placement, and other functions that it can serve in Recommendation 10. In general terms, the board should be permanent, should represent professional excellence on a national scale, and should have facility with issues that have policy ramifications. We see advantages in locating the board outside the government.

The board's role is mainly scientific. It should define the components of risk assessment and describe the scientific basis for each. When it finds general scientific agreement on the proper inference option for a component, it should designate that option in a recommended guideline. When the board finds no general scientific agreement on the available inference options, it should recommend against the use of options that are scientifically unsupportable and comment on the relative strength of the scientific support for the options that remain.*

Agency Adoption

The Committee envisions that the second step in the establishment of guidelines will be in the hands of the

---

*Some members of the Committee believe that the board should also be encouraged in such cases to recommend the option that it judges to have the most scientific support, as long as the board clearly indicates that such choices are based on members' informed scientific judgment, not on general agreement in the scientific community. Other Committee members believe that such recommendations would imply scientific certainty where none exists and thus would result in scientists' improperly recommending policy on the basis of their subjective judgments.

government. The choice of guidelines is, ultimately, the
responsibility of duly elected or appointed public
officials, and public review and comment on the proposed
guidelines should be completed before they are adopted.
The Committee emphasizes that, to be most useful, the
final guidelines should prescribe default options for all
components of risk assessment. Thus, the second step
should further limit the inference options available to
the agencies, even for components in which the board
found that no single option could be chosen on scientific
grounds. In that case, full consideration should be
given to the board's comments on the merit of the scientific support that is available for each option.

It is important that the process result in a timely,
uniform set of inference guidelines to be used by all
agencies. We thus see advantage in coordination of the
agencies' adoption of guidelines by a single, central
authority such as the Office of Science and Technology
Policy, or by a mechanism designated by Congress.

The Committee believes that adopting the guidelines as
established procedures, rather than as formal regulations, would have several important advantages: it would
allow guidelines to be adopted and amended more easily;
it would bind the agencies to adhere to the guidelines
until they were reviewed and revised (thus fostering
predictability and consistency--any agency's failure to
comply with its own guidelines could be noted by independent scientific review panels and could be cited as
grounds for interested parties' legal appeal of an
associated regulatory decision); and it would permit
members of the public to advocate new or alternative
approaches to risk assessment.

Joint risk assessments performed by interagency task
forces should be governed by the guidelines that emerge
from this process.

Uniformity

The Committee has presented its case for uniformity in
guidelines: consistency in the conduct of risk assessment
reduces the appearance of unfair and inconsistent regulatory policies, improves priority-setting among regulators'
programs, increases public understanding, and provides
coherence for those subject to various regulatory authorities. A frequent argument against government-wide guidelines is that different agencies have statutory respon-

sibilities that reflect different social policies and
therefore require different approaches to risk assessment. This argument reflects a misunderstanding of the
purpose of guidelines. An agency would remain free to
incorporate whatever social judgments are embodied in its
mandate when deciding whether and how to regulate. Such
risk management choices can be made independently of and
after the completion of a risk assessment. Thus, two
agencies could use the same risk assessment of a substance, but regulate it differently on the basis of
statutory or policy criteria applied after risk
assessment.

Periodic Review

The scientific basis of risk assessment is evolving
rapidly. Guidelines must continue to evolve to accommodate scientific innovations and theories. By their
very nature, guidelines themselves will help to foster
evolutionary improvements by defining generic principles
of risk assessment and focusing debate and empirical
research on these principles.

Furthermore, new public perceptions of risk occur, and
guidelines will evolve in response to these changes as
well. For example, attitudes about the practicality of
the outright elimination of carcinogenic risk as a regulatory goal have changed in the last decade. New methods
of quantitative risk assessment have developed, and public
discussions have increasingly focused on that field.
These changes can be expected to continue, so regular
periodic review of guidelines appears to be essential.
Such review should follow the same procedures recommended
for the initial guidelines, including ultimate agency
adoption after public comment.

RECOMMENDATION 8

The Committee recommends that guidelines initially be
developed, adopted, and applied for assessment of cancer
risks. Consideration of other types of health effects
should follow. It may not yet be feasible to draw up as
complete a set of inference guidelines for some other
health effects. For these, defining the extent of scientific knowledge and uncertainties and suggesting methods
for dealing with uncertainties would constitute a useful
first step.

The Committee believes that guidelines for carcinogenic risk assessment should be drawn up first, both because cancer is perceived as a major public-health hazard and because there is considerable experience with carcinogenic risk assessment from which to draw. Several guideline documents for carcinogenic risk assessment have already been produced, and review of these documents and of their history should provide a useful point of departure.

However, the other health effects that result from exposure to hazardous substances are equally amenable to prevention by regulatory action. Guidelines are desirable for these types of effects, which include mutagenicity, reproductive and teratogenic effects, neurotoxicity, and behavioral changes. Less information (and, in some cases, less knowledge of causal mechanisms) is usually available on these effects. In fact, in some situations where the knowledge base is less adequate than in cancer, stipulated methods for handling scientific uncertainty may be even more important. Risk assessments for cancer are likely more frequently to engage the problems of evaluating data on exposure of experimental animals, whereas many other health effects will require greater reliance on epidemiologic evidence.

The Committee believes that the absence of guidelines for a health effect is not a justification for agency failure to perform risk assessments or to regulate on a case-by-case basis.

RECOMMENDATION 9

Agencies should develop guidelines for exposure assessment. Because of diverse problems in estimating different means of exposure (e.g., through food, drinking water, and consumer products), separate guidelines may be needed for each.

Operating assumptions are needed to estimate exposures when direct measurements cannot be obtained. Examples of cases in which such estimates would be important are the projection of exposure to new chemicals and determination of the exposure reduction that would result from implementation of a particular control option. In only a few narrow cases (e.g., food additives) have general guidelines been developed for exposure assessment.

Although they are no less important than techniques for hazard identification and dose-response assessment, exposure assessment techniques have not been the subject of major scientific debate and scrutiny. For example, if exposure were known more accurately, priority-setting for testing new chemicals or for initiating regulation of one of a group of chemicals could be organized on a more rigorous basis; consideration of both the apparent potency and the estimated exposure would be factored into such decisions.

Exposure assessment guidelines that are uniform across federal programs may not be feasible, because of the diversity of media that must be addressed and the large variation in exposures. Medium-specific exposure models (such as dispersion models for air, water, and soil) are used by programs in the agencies with various degrees of sophistication and validation. Each agency or each program in an agency should develop medium-specific guidelines to stimulate evolutionary improvement, increase consistency and predictability, and isolate the choice among inference options from inappropriate risk management considerations. Two or more programs that deal with a given medium of exposure should use the same guidelines.

Agencies should make their proposed exposure assessment guidelines available for public comment and should subsequently issue final guidelines as established procedures.

A CENTRAL BOARD ON RISK ASSESSMENT METHODS

RECOMMENDATION 10

The Committee recommends to Congress that a Board on Risk Assessment Methods be established to perform the following functions:

• To assess critically the evolving scientific basis of risk assessment and to make explicit the underlying assumptions and policy ramifications of the different inference options in each component of the risk assessment process.
• To draft and periodically to revise recommended inference guidelines for risk assessment for adoption and use by federal regulatory agencies.
• To study agency experience with risk assessment and evaluate the usefulness of the guidelines.
• To identify research needs in the risk assessment field and in relevant underlying disciplines.

To avoid possible misunderstanding of the role of the Board, the Committee stresses the limitations on proposed Board activities. The Board would not perform or review individual risk assessments, nor would it adjudicate disputes arising from regulatory actions related to specific substances. Thus, the Board as envisioned would not perform functions contemplated by the AIHC proposal or H.R. 638. A central board of distinguished expert advisors is not well-suited to such day-to-day responsibilities. Furthermore, we believe strongly that it would be inappropriate to remove such essential analytic functions from the responsible agencies and that it would be wasteful to duplicate agency activities.

The Board would make its contributions through discussion of contending scientific positions, preparation of recommended uniform guidelines, and fostering of advancement of the field. It would fill a need for a prestigious, independent locus of activity for improving the understanding of generic issues in both the scientific basis and the federal practice of risk assessment. Current ad hoc approaches too often color debate on general issues with the implications for particular, often contentious, risk management decisions. We expect that Board activities would improve the scientific performance of the agency processes and, in conjunction with other mechanisms we recommend, achieve greater objectivity and consistency and better public understanding of risk assessment. The Board would be the body to which agencies, agency review panels, and others would turn both for periodic recommendations of guideline revisions and for information on the evolving art of risk assessment.

Board Functions

We foresee four major functions for the Board. The first two, scientific review and development of recommended guidelines, would pursue the process described above for the initial generation of inference guidelines (Recommendation 7). The drafting of guidelines by the Board would ensure that guidelines benefit from the best available scientific knowledge and judgment. After recommended guidelines for a particular health effect were prepared and referred to the agencies for review and adoption, the Board would probably find it useful to continue its activity in the review of scientific developments relevant to risk assessment for that effect.

The Board's third function would involve observation of and research into federal experience with risk assessment generally and review of the usefulness of guidelines. A major purpose would be to acquaint the Board with ways of improving the guidelines in later periodic reviews.

As a fourth function, the Board would identify the key scientific research needs in health risk assessment. Preparation of guidelines would put the Board in an ideal position to understand which of the many inference options needed to cover gaps in scientific understanding are most important and are amenable to study. The policy difficulties in regulating chronic health hazards can be resolved only if uncertainty in the scientific basis of assessments is reduced. Board activities could take such forms as advising funding agencies on research priorities, commissioning survey papers to synthesize recent scientific findings, and sponsoring conferences or special publications on particularly apt scientific questions or on matters that are important to risk assessment, but have been neglected by the scientific community. In addition, the Board's experience would place it in an ideal position to assess whether and how toxicologic research on particular chemicals could be better tailored to the analytic needs of future risk assessors. For example, many current testing procedures were designed for the narrow purpose of hazard identification, and adjustments in these procedures could lead to more definitive dose-response assessments.

The Committee believes that the responsibilities of the Board could be discharged by a group of volunteer experts that convened monthly for 1-2 days.

Organizational Placement

The proper placement of the Board would be crucial to its prospects for success. There are four criteria for identifying appropriate locations: professional excellence, facility with studies having substantial policy ramifications, permanence, and independence.

Professional excellence is important because the Board's recommended guidelines, as well as its other work, should be based on the best available science; the Board should be able to attract the best talent in the nation. Facility with difficult policy issues is important because risk assessment is not a strictly scientific undertaking, and it would be crucial for the Board to conduct its work competently and with full understanding of the policy process. Placement in a permanent, existing organization is advisable because the Board should be able to begin its work quickly and remain stable in order to conduct periodic revisions of guidelines. Independence is needed to provide credibility; work that is suspected of bias will not transcend the current atmosphere of distrust. We see advantages in placing the Board outside the government. In particular, the Board should be able to draw on the widest pool of scientific experts and not be restricted to government scientists; placement in the government might hinder the perception that the Board is free from the policy orientation of the administration in power; and direct involvement by the regulatory agencies themselves could detract from their ability to make regulatory decisions while the guidelines were in preparation.

The Committee has evaluated a number of possible organizational bases for the Board. The National Toxicology Program has had relevant experience with the scientific basis of risk assessment, but it already has major responsibility for coordinating testing of chemicals of interest to regulatory agencies. The Congressional Office of Technology Assessment is another possibility. However, the governance of the Office of Technology Assessment by a board composed of members of Congress could prove a practical impediment to the production of guidelines. Guidelines would clearly have policy ramifications that may be at variance with the established policy positions of OTA board members. The Office of Science and Technology Policy or the Office of Management and Budget could provide government-wide coordination; both are in the Executive Office of the President and are well positioned to ensure agency response and uniform implementation of guidelines and other Board findings. The major disadvantage of location in the Executive Office of the President is the lack of independence and, consequently, the greater likelihood of mixing scientific and policy considerations. All these organizations share the major drawback that they are in the government.

A special-purpose national (or Presidential) commission on risk assessment methods could attract eminent scientists to service and could be designed to balance viewpoints, but would lack permanence and policy experience. Professional societies constitute another class of possible candidates, but they generally have limited familiarity with policy studies.

We conclude that the National Academy of Sciences-
National Research Council meets the four criteria for
placement. The AIHC proposal addressed the same general
concerns that have occupied this Committee and concluded
that the most appropriate locus for the central panel was
in the NAS-NRC. Although we do not concur in the idea of
centralizing the performance of risk assessments, the
arguments presented by the AIHC proposal for the selection
of the NAS-NRC are fully applicable to the question of
the placement of a Board that would address generic scientific issues in risk assessment. We believe that the
Board could best function under NAS-NRC auspices, if the
NAS-NRC agreed to provide them, and would be of great
value in achieving many of the goals that we share with
the authors of the AIHC proposal and of H.R. 638. Current
NAS-NRC procedures for establishing, managing, and issuing
study reports are appropriate for the prospective Board.

Qualifications of Members

We recommend that the Board consist of scientists with
training and experience in the various disciplines
involved in the process of risk assessment, including
biostatistics, toxicology, epidemiology, environmental
engineering, and clinical medicine. Other relevant
fields--such as law, ethics, and the social sciences--
should be included to ensure due appreciation of the
policy context of Board activities. For the same reason,
some members should have familiarity with regulatory
programs. The nomination and selection of members should
be in accordance with established NAS-NRC procedures.
Service might be for staggered 3-year periods.

Sunset Review

The entire concept of the Board and its functions should
be reviewed after approximately 6-8 years.

Background Information
on Committee Members

REUEL A. STALLONES, <u>Chairman,</u> is Dean of the University
of Texas School of Public Health in Houston. Dr.
Stallones is an epidemiologist specializing in studies
of risk factors in cardiovascular disease and is a
member of the Institute of Medicine. He is a past
member of the NRC Board on Toxicology and Environmental Health Hazards and has served on several NRC
committees that evaluated the risks of environmental
pollutants.

MORTON CORN is Director of the Division of Environmental
Health Engineering at the School of Hygiene and Public
Health, The Johns Hopkins University. He specializes
in evaluation and engineering control of airborne
chemical agents in the workplace and the atmosphere.
Dr. Corn served as the Assistant Secretary of Labor
for Occupational Safety and Health from October 1975
to January 1977. He is a member of the Panel of
Experts in Occupational Health of the World Health
Organization and serves on committees of EPA's Science
Advisory Board and the Congressional Office of
Technology Assessment.

KENNY S. CRUMP is President of Science Research Systems,
Inc., a consulting firm specializing in the evaluation
of statistical data and risk assessment. His work on
methods of extrapolating from high to low doses is
used by EPA's Carcinogen Assessment Group. He was
previously with Louisiana Tech University where he was
Professor of Mathematics and Statistics.

J. CLARENCE DAVIES is Executive Vice President of the
Conservation Foundation. He has served on other NRC

committees dealing with regulatory issues, was chairman of the NRC Committee on Principles of Decision Making for Regulating Chemicals in the Environment (1974-1975), and now serves on the Environmental Studies Board. Dr. Davies served for 6 years as a member of the Executive Committee of EPA's Science Advisory Board.

VINCENT P. DOLE is Professor of Medicine at Rockefeller University and conducts research on addictive behavior and metabolic diseases. Dr. Dole is a member of the National Academy of Sciences and has served as an NAS reviewer of a number of risk-related studies.

TED R. I. GREENWOOD is Associate Professor of Political Science at MIT. He has served as a Senior Policy Analyst in the Office of Science and Technology Policy (1977-1979). Dr. Greenwood has written about the problem of nuclear waste disposal and recently completed a monograph on the interaction between knowledge and discretion in regulatory decision-making.

RICHARD A. MERRILL is Dean of the Law School of the University of Virginia. He has been on the Law School faculty since 1969, except for 2 years (1975-1977), when he served as Chief Counsel to the FDA. He recently completed a study of regulatory decision-making on carcinogens for the Administrative Conference of the United States that focused on FDA's regulation of food contaminants, CPSC's regulation of chronic hazards, OSHA's program for workplace carcinogens, and the EPA pesticides program. Dean Merrill is a member of the Institute of Medicine and the NRC Board on Toxicology and Environmental Health Hazards. He teaches food and drug law, environmental health regulation, and administrative law.

FRANKLIN E. MIRER is Director of the Health and Safety Department of the International Union, United Auto Workers. Dr. Mirer, an industrial hygienist and toxicologist, has been with the UAW since 1975. He specializes in issues related to workplace chemical exposures and development of OSHA standards.

D. WARNER NORTH is a Principal with Decision Focus, Inc., a consulting firm specializing in decision analysis, and consulting Associate Professor with the Department

of Engineering-Economic Systems at Stanford University.
Over the last 15 years, Dr. North has carried out
applications of decision analysis and risk assessment
to a variety of public-policy issues. He has participated in three previous NRC studies on air quality and
toxic chemicals. His recent projects include work on
methods for setting priorities and developing a
regulatory strategy for toxic chemicals for the EPA
Office of Toxic Substances. Dr. North has served on
committees of the EPA Science Advisory Board since
1977.

GILBERT S. OMENN is Dean of the School of Public Health
of the University of Washington in Seattle. A
physician and geneticist, Dr. Omenn served in senior
positions in the Office of Science and Technology
Policy and in the Office of Management and Budget
(1977-1981). He is a member of the Institute of
Medicine. At OSTP, he was concerned with federal
decision-making for public-health risks and was
coauthor of a paper on the process for making such
decisions. Before returning to the University of
Washington, Dr. Omenn was a Fellow at the Brookings
Institution, where he analyzed EPA's 1979 decision to
revise the national ambient air quality standard for
photochemical oxidants (measured as ozone).

JOSEPH V. RODRICKS is a Principal with ENVIRON
Corporation, a Washington, D.C., consulting firm
specializing in risks related to exposure to toxic
substances. Dr. Rodricks, a biochemist, was with the
FDA for 15 years (1965-1980). While at FDA, he served
as Deputy Associate Commissioner and as chairman of an
interagency work group on risk assessment that developed guidelines for member agencies to follow for
determining risks associated with exposure to carcinogenic chemicals. Dr. Rodricks is a member of the NRC
Board on Toxicology and Environmental Health Hazards
and a Diplomate of the American Board of Toxicology.

PAUL SLOVIC is a psychologist at Decision Research in
Eugene, Oregon. His research interests are related to
human judgment in decision-making, with special
emphasis on perception of risk, and he is coauthor of
a book on the concept of acceptable risk. Dr. Slovic
has served as a consultant to FDA, NSF, the National
Institute of Mental Health, and the Nuclear Regulatory

Commission. He has been a council member of the
Society for Risk Analysis and is President-elect of
that organization.

H. MICHAEL D. UTIDJIAN is Corporate Medical Director at
the American Cyanamid Company. Dr. Utidjian has been
active in occupational medicine since 1961. Before
gaining his current position, he was a Staff Scientist
at Stanford Research Institute and served as a
consultant to NIOSH. He also served as Associate
Corporate Medical Director at Union Carbide.

ELIZABETH WEISBURGER is Assistant Director for Chemical
Carcinogenesis at the National Cancer Institute. Dr.
Weisburger, a toxicologist/oncologist, has been at NCI
for 33 years and was involved in initial NCI decisions
on establishing its bioassay program and determining
which compounds to test.

APPENDIX B
Bibliography

A. GUIDELINES AND POLICY FOR RISK ASSESSMENT

Albert, R. E., R. Train, and E. Anderson. Rationale
Developed by EPA for the Assessment of Carcinogenic
Risks. Journal of the NCI Vol. 58, No. 5, May 1977,
pp. 1537-1541.

Calkins, D. R., R. L. Dixon, C. R. Gerber, D. Zarin, and
G. S. Omenn. Identification, Characterization and
Control of Potential Human Carcinogens: A Framework
for Federal Decision-Making. Journal of the NCI Vol.
64, No. 1, January 1980, pp. 169-176.

Consumer Product Safety Commission. Interim Policy and
Procedure for Classifying, Evaluating, and Regulating
Carcinogens in Consumer Products. Federal Register
Vol. 43, No. 114, June 13, 1978, pp. 25658-25665.

Department of Labor, Occupational Safety and Health
Administration. Identification, Classification, and
Regulation of Potential Occupational Carcinogens.
Federal Register Book 2 of 2, Vol. 45, No. 15, January
22, 1980, pp. 5001-5296.

Environmental Protection Agency. Health Risk and
Economic Impact Assessments of Suspected Carcinogens:
Interim Procedures and Guidelines. Federal Register
Vol. 41, No. 102, May 25, 1976, pp. 21402-21405.

Environmental Protection Agency. Mutagenicity Risk
Assessments; Proposed Guidelines. Federal Register
Vol. 45, No. 221, November 13, 1980, pp. 74984-74988.

Food and Drug Administration. Chemical Compounds in Food
Producing Animals: Criteria and Procedures for
Evaluating Assays for Carcinogenic Residues. Federal
Register Vol. 44, No. 55, May 20, 1979, pp.
17070-17114.

International Agency for Research on Cancer. General
    Principles for Evaluating the Carcinogenic Risk of
    Chemicals. In Evaluation of the Carcinogenic Risk of
    Chemicals to Humans. IARC, Lyon, France, Vols. 1-29,
    1972-1982.
Interagency Regulatory Liaison Group. Work Group on Risk
    Assessment. Scientific Bases for Identification of
    Potential Carcinogens and Estimation of Risks.
    Journal of the NCI Vol. 63, No. 1, July 1979, 25 pp.
    and Abstract.
March of Dimes Birth Defects Foundation. Guidelines for
    Studies of Human Populations Exposed to Mutagenic and
    Reproductive Hazards; Proceedings of Conference.
    Washington, D.C., January 26-27, 1981, 163 pp.
National Academy of Sciences. Committee for a Study on
    Saccharin and Food Safety Policy. Food Safety
    Policy: Scientific and Social Considerations.
    NAS-NRC, March 1979.
National Academy of Sciences. Committee on the
    Biological Effects of Ionizing Radiations. The
    Effects on Populations of Exposure to Low Levels of
    Ionizing Radiation. NAS-NRC, 1980, 638 pp.
National Cancer Advisory Board. General Criteria for
    Assessing the Evidence of Carcinogenecity of Chemical
    Substances. Report of the Subcommittee on
    Environmental Carcinogenesis, NCAB. Journal of the
    NCI Vol. 58, No. 2, February 1977, pp. 461-465.
State of California, Health and Welfare Agency. Carcino-
    gen Identification Policy: A Statement of Science as
    a Basis of Policy; Section 2: Methods for Estimating
    Cancer Risks from Exposure to Carcinogens. October
    1982.
U.S. Regulatory Council. Statement on Regulation of
    Chemical Carcinogens: Policy and Request for Public
    Comments. Federal Register Part IV, Vol. 44, No. 202,
    October 17, 1979, pp. 60038-60049.

B. SUGGESTIONS FOR PROCEDURAL REFORM

Albert, R. A. Toward a More Uniform Federal Strategy for
    the Assessment and Regulation of Carcinogens. Report
    to the Office of Technology Assessment, 1980.
American Industrial Health Council. AIHC Proposal for a
    Science Panel (mimeo), March 12, 1981, 9 pp. and
    Appendix, AIHC Recommended Framework for Identifying
    Carcinogens and Regulating Them in Manufacturing
    Situations, October 11, 1979, 11 pp.

American Industrial Health Council. Comparative Analysis of H.R. 6521 (Wampler Bill) and Science Panel Proposal, March 3, 1980.

American Industrial Health Council. Critical Evaluation of Proposals by the AIHC to Strengthen the Scientific Base for Regulatory Decisions; Report of the Scientific Workshop (mimeo), August 1982, 6 pp.

American Industrial Health Council. Proposals for Improving the Science Base for Chronic Health Hazard Decision-Making, December 2, 1981, 29 pp. and Appendixes.

Banks, R. The Science Court Proposal in Retrospect: A Literature Review and Case Study. Critical Reviews in Environmental Control Vol. 10, August 1980, pp. 95-131.

Barr, J. T., D. H. Hughes, and R. C. Barnard. The Use of Risk Assessment in Regulatory Decision Making: Time for a Review. Regulatory Toxicology and Pharmacology Vol. 1, 1981, pp. 264-276.

Bazelon, D. L. Risk and Responsibility. Science Vol. 205, July 20, 1979, pp. 277-280.

Boffey, P. M. Science Court: High Officials Back Test of Controversial Concept. Science Vol. 194, October 8, 1976, pp. 167-169.

Deisler, P. F., Jr. Dealing with Industrial Health Risks: A Step-Wise, Goal-Oriented Concept. In Risk in the Technological Society, Hohenemser and Kasperson, eds. Westview Press, 1981.

Food Safety Council. Social and Economic Committee. A New Approach: Principles and Processes for Making Food Safety Decisions. FSC, 1981, 103 pp. plus Appendixes.

Food Safety Council. A Proposed Food Safety Evaluation Process: Final Report of Board of Trustees. FSC, June 1982, 142 pp.

General Accounting Office. Improving the Scientific and Technical Information Available to the EPA in Its Decision-making Process. Report CED-79-115, September 1979, 60 pp.

Gori, G. B. Regulation of Cancer-Causing Substances: Utopia or Reality. Chemical and Engineering News September 6, 1982, pp. 25-32.

Gori, G. B. The Regulation of Carcinogenic Hazards. Science Vol. 208, April 18, 1980, pp. 256-261.

H.R. 638 (Wampler Bill). National Science Council Act of 1981. Introduced January 8, 1981.

H.R. 6159 (Ritter Bill). Risk Analysis Research and Demonstration Act of 1982. Introduced April 26, 1982.

Kantrowitz, A. Controlling Technology Democratically.
  American Scientist Vol. 63, 1975, pp. 505-509.
Kantrowitz, A. Proposal for an Institution for
  Scientific Judgment. Science Vol. 156, May 12, 1967,
  pp. 763-764.
Markey, H. T. Testimony to the Subcommittee on Science
  Research and Technology, 1979. In Risk/Benefit
  Analysis in the Legislative Process. U.S. Government
  Printing Office, Washington, D.C., 1979.
Martin, J. Procedures for Decision Making Under
  Conditions of Scientific Uncertainty: The Science
  Court Proposal. Harvard Journal of Legislation Vol.
  16, Spring 1979, pp. 443-511.
National Academy of Sciences. Committee on Environmental
  Decision Making. Decision Making in the Environmental
  Protection Agency. NAS-NRC, 1977, 250 pp.
National Academy of Sciences. Committee on Food
  Protection, Food and Nutrition Board. Risk
  Assessment/Safety Evaluation of Food Chemicals.
  NAS-NRC, 1980, 36 pp.
National Academy of Sciences. Committee on Prototype
  Explicit Analyses for Pesticides. Regulating
  Pesticides. NAS-NRC, 1980, 237 pp.
National Academy of Sciences. Committee on Toxicology.
  Principles and Procedures for Evaluating the Toxicity
  of Household Substances. NAS-NRC, 1977, 130 pp.
National Academy of Sciences. Environmental Studies
  Board/Committee on Toxicology. Principles for
  Evaluating Chemicals in the Environment. NAS-NRC,
  1975.
Ramo, S. Regulation of Technical Activities: A New
  Approach. Science Vol. 213, Aug. 21, 1981, pp.
  837-842.
Rowe, W. D. Regulation of Toxic Chemicals Within the
  Limits of Knowledge. Report submitted to the Office
  of Technology Assessment, 1980.
S. 1442 (Hatch Bill). Food Safety Amendments of 1981.
  Introduced June 25, 1981.
Squire, R. A. Ranking Animal Carcinogens: A Proposed
  Regulatory Approach. Science Vol. 214, 1981, pp.
  877-880.
Toxic Substances Strategy of Committee. Report to the
  President: Toxic Chemicals and Public Protection.
  U.S. Government Printing Office, Washington, D.C.,
  1980.
U.S. House of Representatives. Omnibus Budget
  Reconciliation Act of 1981: Conference Report.
  Report 97-208, July 1981, pp. 383-384, 881-883.

U.S. House of Representatives. Committee on Agriculture. The National Science Council Act, June 1981.

U.S. House of Representatives. Committee on Science and Technology. Risk Analysis Research and Demonstration Act of 1982. Report No. 97-625, June 24, 1982.

Wessel, M. R. Science and Conscience. Columbia University Press, 1980, 140 pp.

C. SCIENTIFIC AND POLICY BASIS OF RISK ASSESSMENT

Ames, B. N. Identifying Environmental Chemicals Causing Mutations and Cancer. Science Vol. 204, May 22, 1979, pp. 587-593.

Anderson, E. L. Quantitative Methods in Use in the United States to Assess Cancer Risk. Paper presented at the Workshop on Quantitative Estimation of Risk to Human Health from Chemicals, Rome, Italy, July 12, 1982.

Anderson, E. L. Uses of Quantitative Risk Assessment by EPA (mimeo). Prepublication draft, 18 pp.

Ashford, N. A., E. M. Zolt, D. Hattis, J. I. Natz, G. R. Heaton, and W. C. Priest. Evaluating Chemical Regulations: Trade-off Analysis and Impact Assessment for Environmental Decision-Making (mimeo). MIT Center for Policy Alternatives, 1979.

Baram, M. S. Cost-Benefit Analysis: An Inadequate Basis for Health, Safety, and Environmental Regulatory Decisionmaking. Ecology Law Quarterly Vol. 8, No. 3, 1980, pp. 473-531.

Campbell, G., D. Cohan, and D. W. North. The Application of Decision Analysis to Toxic Substances: Proposed Methodology and Two Case Studies. Prepared for EPA by Decision Focus Incorporated, 1981.

Cornfield, J. Carcinogenic Risk Assessment. Science Vol. 198, November 18, 1977, pp. 693-699.

Crandall, R. W., and L. B. Lave, eds. The Scientific Basis of Health and Safety Regulation. Brookings Institution, 1981, 309 pp.

Crouch, E., and R. Wilson. Interspecies Comparison of Carcinogenic Potency. Journal of Toxicology and Environmental Health Vol. 5, 1979, pp. 1095-1118, plus Appendixes.

Crouch, E., and R. Wilson. Regulation of Carcinogens. Risk Analysis Vol. 1, 1981, pp. 47-57; discussion pp. 59-66.

Crump, K. S.   An Improved Procedure for Low-Dose
    Carcinogenic Risk Assessment from Animal Data.
    Journal of Environmental Pathology and Toxicology Vol.
    5, No. 4, 1983.
Crump, K. S.   Dose-Response Problems in Carcinogenesis.
    Biometrics Vol. 35, March 1979, pp. 157-167.
Crump, K. S., D. Hoel, C. Langley, and R. Peto.   Funda-
    mental Carcinogenic Processes and Their Implications
    for Low Dose Risk Assessment.   Cancer Research Vol 36,
    September 1979, pp. 2973-2979.
Crump, K. S.   The Scientific Basis for Health Risk
    Assessment.   Presentation at the seminar sponsored by
    George Washington University Graduate Program in
    Science, Technology, and Public Policy and by the EPA,
    Washington, D.C., March 3, 1982.
Devoret, R.   Bacterial Tests for Potential Carcinogens.
    Scientific American Vol. 241, No. 2, August 1979, pp.
    40-49.
Doll, R., and R. Peto.   The Causes of Cancer: Quantita-
    tive Estimates of Avoidable Risks of Cancer in the
    United States Today.   Journal of the NCI Vol. 66. No.
    6, June 1981, pp. 1191-1308.
Doniger, D., R. Liroff, and N. Dean.   An Analysis of Past
    Federal Efforts to Control Toxic Substances.   Report
    to CEQ by the Environmental Law Institute, July 20,
    1978, 71 pp.
Dower, R. C., and D. Maldonado.   An Overview: Assessing
    the Benefits of Environmental Health and Safety
    Regulations.   U.S. Regulatory Council, 1981, 34 pp.
Gelpe, M. R., and A. D. Tarlock.   The Uses of Scientific
    Information in Environmental Decisionmaking.   Southern
    California Law Review Vol. 48, 1974, pp. 371-427.
Greenwood, T.   Assessment of the Role of Science and
    Technology in Standard-Setting by Two Federal
    Regulatory Agencies.   Report to OSTP, March 1, 1981,
    308 pp.
Greenwood, T.   Knowledge and Descretion in Regulation
    (forthcoming).
Fischhoff, B., S. Lichtenstein, P. Slovic, S. L. Derby,
    and R. L. Keeney.   Acceptable Risk.   Cambridge
    University Press, 1981, 185 pp.
Flamm, W. G.   U.S. Approaches to Regulatory Carcinogens
    and Mutagens in Food (mimeo).   Address to the National
    Cancer Institute of Canada and Toxicology Forum
    Conference, Vancouver, August 13, 1981.
Gaylor, D. W.   The ED_{01} Study.   Summary and Conclusion.
    Journal of Environmental Pathology and Toxicology Vol.
    3, 1979, pp. 179-183.

Higgins, I. T. T. Importance of Epidemiological Studies
Relating to Hazards of Food and Environment. British
Medical Bulletin Vol. 31, No. 3, 1975, pp. 230-235.

Hoel, D. G., D. W. Gaylor, R. L. Kirschstein, U.
Saffiotti, and M. A. Schneiderman. Estimation of
Risks of Irreversible Delayed Toxicity. Journal of
Toxicology and Environmental Health Vol. 7, 1975, pp.
133-151.

Howard, R. A., J. E. Matheson, and D. W. North. Decision
Analysis for Environmental Protection Decisions. SRI,
June 1977, 67 pp.

Karch, N. J. Explicit Criteria and Principles for
Identifying Carcinogens: A Focus of Controversy and
EPA. Volume IIa, Case Studies, National Academy of
Sciences, 1977, pp. 119-206.

Lave, L., and T. Romer. A Survey of Safety Levels in
Federal Regulation. Nuclear Regulatory Commission
Rep. NUREG/CR-2226, June 1981, 46 pp.

Leape, J. P. Quantitative Risk Assessment in Regulation
of Environmental Carcinogens. Harvard Environmental
Law Review Vol. 4, 1980, pp. 86-116.

Leventhal, H. Environmental Decisionmaking and the Role
of the Courts. University of Pennsylvania Law Review
Vol. 122, January 1974, pp. 509-555.

Lowrance, W. W. Of Acceptable Risk: Science and The
Determination of Safety. William Kaufmann, Inc., Los
Altos, Calif., 1976, 180 pp.

Mantel, N., and M. Schneiderman. Estimating "Safe"
Levels, A Hazardous Undertaking. Cancer Research Vol.
35, June 1975, pp. 1379-1386.

McGarity, T. O. Substantive and Procedural Discretion
in Administrative Resolution of Science Policy
Questions: Regulating Carcinogens in EPA and OSHA.
Georgetown Law Journal Vol. 67, 1979, pp. 729-810.

Merrill, R. A. CPSC Regulation of Cancer Risks in
Consumer Products. Virginia Law Review Vol. 67, 1981,
p. 1261.

Merrill, R. A. FDA Regulation Environmental Contamination of Food. Virginia Law Review Vol. 66, 1980, p.
1357.

Merrill, R. A. Federal Regulation of Cancer-Causing
Chemicals. (mimeo). Report to the Administrative
Conference of the United States. April 1, 1982.

Munro, I. C., and D. R. Krewski. Risk Assessment and
Regulatory Decisionmaking. Food and Cosmetic
Toxicology Vol. 19, 1981, pp. 549-560.

National Academy of Sciences. Committee on Risk and Decison-Making. Risk and Decision Making: Perspectives and Research. NAS-NRC, 1982 68 pp.

National Academy of Sciences. Governing Board; Committee on the Assessment of Risks. The Handling of Risk Assessments in NRC Reports (mimeo.). March 1981, 27 pp.

Nicholson, W. J., ed. Management of Assessed Risk for Carcinogens. New York Academy of Sciences, 1981, 301 pp.

Nisbet, I. C. T., and N. J. Karch. Chemical Hazards to Human Reproduction. Noyes Data, Park Ridge, N.J., 1983.

Office of Technology Assessment. Assessment of Technologies for Determining Cancer Risks from the Environment. Office of Technology Assessment, June 1981, 240 pp.

Oak Ridge National Laboratory/Environmental Protection Agency. Assessment of Risks to Human Reproduction and to Development of Human Conceptus from Exposure to Environmental Substances. ORNL/EIS-197, EPA/9-82-001, February 1982, 158 pp.

Omenn, G. S. Risk Assessment and Environmental Policy-Making: An Overview. Presentation at the seminar sponsored by George Washington University Graduate Program in Science, Technology, and Public Policy and by the EPA, Washington, D.C., January 27, 1982.

Rall, D. P. The Role of Laboratory Animal Studies in Estimating Carcinogenic Risks for Man. Address to IARC Symposium, "Carcinogenic Risks-Strategies for Intervention," Lyon, France, 1977, 12 pp.

Ricci, P. F., and L. S. Molton. Risk and Benefit in Environmental Law. Science Vol. 214, December 4, 1981, pp. 1096-1100.

Rodricks, J. V., and R. G. Tardiff. Biological Bases for Risk Assessment. Paper presented at the International Conference on Safety Evaluation and Regulation of Chemicals, Session 2: State of the Art of Safety Evaluation, Boston, Mass., February 24-26, 1982.

Rowe, W. D. An Anatomy of Risk. Wiley-Interscience, New York, 1977.

Samuels, S. W. Determination of Cancer Risk in a Democracy. Annals of the New York Academy of Sciences Vol. 271, 1976, pp. 421-430.

Thomas, L., S. J. Farber, R. A. Doherty, A. Koppas, and A. A. Upton. Report of the Governor's Panel to Review Scientific Studies and the Development of Public

Policy on Problems Resulting from Hazardous Wastes (mimeo). New York State, October 1980, 33 pp.

Van Ryzin, J. Quantitative Risk Assessment. _Journal of Occupational Medicine_ Vol. 22, No. 5, May 1980, pp. 321-326.

Weinberg, A. M. Science and Trans-Science. _Minerva_ No. 10, 1972, pp. 202-222.

Weisburger, J. H., and G. M. Williams. Carcinogen Testing: Current Problems and New Approaches. _Science_ Vol. 214, October 23, 1980 pp. 401-407.

D. BIBLIOGRAPHIES

Krewski, D., and C. Brown. Carcinogenic Risk Assessment: A Guide to the Literature. _Biometrics_ Vol. 37, June 1981, pp. 353-366.

Tardiff, R. G. Extrapolation: High to Low Doses (mimeo). National Academy of Sciences, September 1981, 5 pp.

Tardiff, R. G. Extrapolation: High to Low Doses Combined with Laboratory Animals to Humans (mimeo). National Academy of Sciences, October 1981, 6 pp.

Tardiff, R. G. Extrapolation. Laboratory Animals to Humans (mimeo). National Academy of Sciences, October 1981, 6 pp.

(Photocopies of the collected working papers of the
Committee on the Institutional Means for Assessment of
Risks to Public Health are available from the National
Academy Press, 2101 Constitution Avenue, NW, Washington,
DC 20418)

CASE STUDY: CPSC'S RISK ASSESSMENT FOR FORMALDEHYDE
     William M. Stigliani

CASE STUDY: NITRITE
     Catherine L. St. Hilaire

CASE STUDY: ASBESTOS RISK ASSESSMENTS BY OSHA/NIOSH
     AND EPA
     William M. Stigliani

AN ANATOMY OF RISK ASSESSMENT
     Lawrence E. McCray

CURRENT FEDERAL PRACTICE IN RISK ASSESSMENT
     Lawrence E. McCray and Robert I. Field